HOLISTIC CHEMOTHERAPY
Combining Holistic Methods with Conventional Treatment Plans

Copyright © 2017

Tami Dickerson, M.H.
Front Cover design: Kevin E. Rouse

Although the information contained in this book is evidence-based it is not intended to replace your physician's advice. Be sure to have a discussion with your physician(s) before making any changes in any of your treatment plans.

TABLE OF CONTENTS

When I am afraid, I will trust in You.
– Psalm 56:3 (CSB)*

Chapter 1
FINDING A GOOD HOLISTIC PRACTITIONER

It is common knowledge that chemotherapy is a challenging experience; therefore many patients seek non-conventional therapies with hopes of finding treatments which are less harsh yet still effective. These therapies are often referred to as alternative, complementary, or holistic medicine. Many people do not realize there are differences in these methods, therefore I will give a brief explanation here:

- ALTERNATIVE MEDICINE: This is exactly what it sounds like – a method which is alternative to conventional medicine. An example of this would be when a patient uses the inhaled vapors of eucalyptus oil to clear a stuffy nose instead of using an over-the-counter cold remedy.

- COMPLEMENTARY MEDICINE a.k.a. INTEGRATIVE MEDICINE: These are non-conventional methods which are used alongside conventional medicine, therefore they complement conventional medicine. An example of this would be drinking ginger tea to counteract the nausea caused by a chemotherapy treatments.

- HOLISTIC MEDICINE: Alternative, complementary, and conventional medicine all treat the physical body; in contrast, holistic medicine goes a few steps further and treats the whole person: body, *and* mind, *and* spirit. An example of holistic therapy may include using guided imagery sessions to alleviate anxiety during cancer treatment.

Oftentimes these three categories may overlap. For example, the patient using ginger tea to counteract nausea instead of using anti-nausea medications is following a method that is both complimentary *and* alternative. Because of this overlap I will refer to alternative, complementary, and holistic methods under the umbrella term "*holistic*," and those who are holistic-based professionals will be referenced as "*practitioner(s)*." In contrast, professionals who practice *conventional* medicine will be referred to as doctors or physicians unless otherwise noted.[1]

The United States government requires specific categories of holistic practitioners to be formally educated and licensed in order to legally practice their trade, such as chiropractors and osteopaths. Other forms of holistic medicine such as massage therapists, music therapists, acupuncturists, and practitioners of Traditional Chinese Medicine must be either licensed or certified depending upon location of practice. Naturopathic Practitioners, formally titled as "Naturopathic Doctors, " are allowed to be licensed only in specific locations.[2]

---

1   The one exception is the title "Naturopathic Doctor", which is the official title of certain holistic practitioners.

2   As of this writing these locations are: Alaska, Arizona, California, Colorado, Connecticut, District of Columbia, Hawaii, Kansas, Maine, Maryland, Massachusetts, Minnesota, Montana, New

The United States government does *not* require the formal education or licensing of other practitioners such as herbalists, homeopaths, aromatherapists, Ayurvedic practitioners, guided imagery therapists and, in most places, naturopathic doctors. When it comes to these non-licensed practitioners you must keep certain things in mind when choosing the practitioner:

- Non-licensed practitioners are not legally allowed to diagnose health conditions, treat health conditions, or prescribe substances for health conditions as these are viewed as felony practicing medicine without a license and felony dispensing drugs without a license. However, non-licensed practitioners *can* legally *educate* clients regarding their physician-diagnosed conditions, *educate* them on which holistic methods are known to be most appropriate for their needs, and *educate* them on the correct ways to use those methods.

- Oftentimes a non-licensed practitioner may carry a legal license/certification for another holistic discipline. For example, although Ayurvedic medicine[3] is a non-licensed practice in itself an Ayurvedic practitioner may be a licensed massage therapist or a certified midwife, therefore he or she can legally treat you within the parameters of massage therapy or midwifery as a licensed professional.

- Non-licensed practitioners must refer to their customers as clients, not patients. They cannot refer to themselves as a "doctor" or "nurse" unless they are already legally licensed as such in their locations of practice.

- A naturopathic doctor (N.D.) who is licensed in one location but practices in a non-licensing location cannot legally operate as a *licensed* practitioner when working in the non-licensed location. In other words, an N. D. licensed in the state of Kansas cannot practice as a *licensed* professional in the neighboring state of Missouri even if the patient's state border is literally across the street from the Kansas practice. This means the N.D. cannot diagnose health problems, treat health issues, or prescribe treatments while examining the client in his own home in Missouri across the street – the client must come across the street to the Kansas-based practice instead.

- Non-licensed practices are not covered by health insurance, therefore your consultations with them will be an out-of-pocket expense for you. However, if your practitioner does hold a license or certification in some other discipline (such as midwifery, massage therapy, etc.) the health insurance may pay for some of the treatments. Be sure to ask questions regarding your health insurance coverage first so that you are not unpleasantly surprised.

Hampshire, North Dakota, Oregon, Pennsylvania, Utah, Vermont, Washington, Puerto Rico, and the United States Virgin Islands.

3   Also known as "Ayurveda"; an ancient form of traditional Indian medicine based in Hindu belief.

When you seek out holistic practitioners you need to be careful of whom you sign on with. Just as you expect your conventional doctor to have a qualified education in order to treat you, you should expect your holistic practitioners (licensed and non-licensed) to be likewise qualified. Be very careful to avoid those who are self-taught or who insist on using methods which have not been scientifically verified.

All schools who educate *licensed* or *certified* practitioners must be accredited by the United States Department of Education; the practitioners must also pass all legal board exams that may be required for their profession before they can practice. Make sure your licensed professional has all of his or her credentials. If your practitioner was educated abroad you should be sure to check that he or she has a valid license or certification to practice in the United States.

As for schools which educate *non-licensed* professionals, these are not required by law to be accredited, and most which are accredited are not accredited through the United States Department of Education. This alternative accreditation is not automatically a deal-breaker as there are schools with alternative accreditations which are very good. Here is what you need to be aware of when looking at a non-licensed practitioner's credentials:

- The self-taught practitioners are the least reliable simply because you do not know what was actually learned. Avoid them. If, instead, he or she was taught by a holistic school this depends upon the quality of education the school offers. Time to investigate the school as follows:

- Check the school's website and see what kinds of classes, materials, and classwork its students are required to complete. Does it require class participation, assignments, homework and tests, or is it a "diploma mill" which simply offers a degree or diploma with little or no classwork? And just so you are aware, an *online* school should also require class participation and assignments and tests; it should be no different.[4]

- Also look for the school's accreditation: It is accredited? By whom? Also, check to see its rating with the Better Business Bureau – be sure the school does not have multiple complaints lodged against it.

- If you are not comfortable with the practitioner's level of education, *find another practitioner*. It is not rude to seek someone else; this is *your* health, it is your right to find someone competent and properly educated.

---

4 Good online schools will give students access to their professors through dedicated site links, require the completion of assignments and tests that are usually submitted through on-site links; provide educational books and media, and allow for class participation through dedicated chat, discussion forums, etc.

Another important thing to consider is your practitioner's basis of therapy. Just as you would expect your doctors to recommend treatments based on valid scientific evidence you should likewise expect your holistic practitioners to base their therapies on legitimate scientific evidence. Cancer is an aggressive disease; you do not have time to chase therapies that are backed only by testimonials from unverifiable "former patients" or anecdotal evidence. No matter how sincere or professional a practitioner may seem, you need to rely on how scientifically *proven* the therapy actually is – which studies support the claims?

Avoid practitioners who actively discourage you from using conventional medicine to treat your cancer. Qualified practitioners will welcome the use of conventional medicine in tandem with the holistic therapies because they know that holistic therapies *alone* are not enough to beat cancer. When it comes to fighting cancer holistic methods are best employed as *synchronized therapy* to boost the effectiveness of the conventional treatments. For example, medical science has shown that heat therapy can weaken cancer cells and make them more vulnerable to chemotherapy medications. Although you would not want to use heat therapy *alone* to treat your cancer, you would certainly want to consider adding it alongside your conventional treatment to boost the effectiveness of your chemotherapy.

Another thing that must be mentioned is that you will probably come across some unconventional cancer "therapies" with strong anecdotal evidence that these work. Keep in mind that *anecdotal* evidence is not proven science, and therefore should not be viewed as solid evidence in favor of a therapy or treatment. I strongly advise that you do not waste your time or money on treatments that have no scientific backing. If you come across treatments which have weak or contradictory scientific evidence then I suggest you speak with your oncologist,[5] in detail, regarding the treatment before you decide. Avoid practitioners who pressure you to start therapy without speaking with your oncologist first.

You also want to consider the practitioner's fee schedule. Holistic practitioners should not be charging exorbitant fees for their services. Granted, some holistic methods may have a wide range of fees per appointment depending upon where the practice is located (more affluent areas tend to charge higher rates). Take your location into consideration when investigating your practitioner's fees. If a practitioner insists on charging a very high fee due to claims of product scarcity or distinctiveness of therapy take your business elsewhere, it is a scam. And keep in mind that successful scammers tend to come across as warm, inviting, and legitimate as genuine practitioners – do not let their demeanor fool you.

Another important item to consider is that you should be concerned if your practitioner is using "secret" methods or formulas without giving you specific information. It is *your* health and there should be *nothing* secret about your own treatments or therapies. Since it is advisable that you inform your oncologist about any holistic therapies you may be using a good practitioner knows that you must be aware of any ingredients, methods, and processes being used in order to ensure these do not interfere with your conventional treatments. Therefore, if a practitioner offers

---

5   Oncologist = The licensed doctor specializing in the treatment of cancer.

you a special blend of herbs or powders, performs any kind of energy-based therapy (heat, ultraviolet light, sound therapy, etc.), offers aromatherapy treatments, etc. be sure he or she tells you exactly what you are being offered so you can properly discuss it with your oncologist. Any practitioner who resists giving you this information for any reason is a fraud and should be dropped immediately.

One last thing I should mention is that it would be wise for you to check the cleanliness of the practice. A good, educated practitioner understands the importance of a clean and hygienic practice for the sake of patient health. People who seek out holistic practitioners are usually people with health problems. Therefore, a worthy practitioner will care enough about patients' well-being to keep the clinic and office space as clean and germ-free as possible. You should expect the place to look as clean and neat as a doctor's office or a conventional clinic room. Look around, see if there are any unhygienic materials lying around in the open: Soiled linens, loose tissues, rags, etc. Are the floors and sinks kept clean? Does all of the equipment, trash, and soiled items have designated places? Do the employees of the place practice good hand washing between clients? If the practitioner uses needles look to see if used needles are disposed of in rigid plastic containers ("sharps containers") and make sure the practitioner is using single-use disposables. If the place looks shabby, unkempt, or dirty, go elsewhere.

In short, when deciding on a holistic practitioner it is important to look into his or her credentials, basis of treatment, philosophy of healing, and hygienic standards. Although you may be worried about your cancer you do not need to make the mistake of wasting your valuable time and money on incompetent practitioners. The sad fact is that many people want so much to believe in a cure that they oftentimes fall victim to unqualified practitioners' promises and testimonials. Cases in point:

- *Dr. Christine Daniels* was a licensed medical doctor and Pentecostal minister who claimed her "cancer cure, " made of sunscreen preservatives, beef extract flavoring, and other ingredients, had up to an 80% cure rate, charging victims up to $100,000 for six months of treatment. She even went so far as to throw a "cured" party for one of her patients who died of the disease shortly afterward. In 2013 Daniels was sentenced to fourteen years in prison for fraud, tax evasion, and witness tampering.

- *Dr. Robert O. Young*, an unlicensed naturopathic doctor educated through an online holistic school,[6] treated cancer patients based on the unscientific idea that cancer is caused by excess acids in the body; he regularly charged $50,000 or more per treatment. He was well-known for convincing patients to avoid chemotherapy and other conventional treatments. His most famous victim was a 50 year old patient named Kim Tinkham. After accepting his treatments she was convinced that she was cured, and even appeared on the

---

6 He earned his degree through the now-defunct Clayton College of Natural Health, which was a holistic school that suddenly closed in 2010. None of the states which license naturopathic doctors have ever accepted naturopathic doctor credentials from Clayton College.

Oprah Winfrey show to praise Dr. Young's treatments. However, in 2010 at age 53, Kim Tinkham died of the very cancer she was told she was cured of. In 2014 Dr. Young was arrested and charged with practicing medicine without a license, and fraud.

- *Vincent Gammill* posed as a doctor and sold bags of dirt, dangerous chemicals and expired medications as cancer cures while charging patients $2,000 per consultation. Gammill was arrested when a victim became suspicious of his methods and turned him in. In 2015 he was charged with practicing medicine without a license and dispensing medications without a license

- *Peter Adeniji* sold his special cancer-curing herbal mixtures for $1,200 per bottle while denouncing conventional cancer treatments. He was turned in by a victim who spent six-thousand dollars on his phony treatments just to have her cancer continually grow. In 2016 Adeniji was arrested and charged with operating a medical practice without a license; dispensing drugs without a license, and fraud.

These are but a scant few of the many fraudulent holistic "healers" that are revealed in the news on a regular basis. Take note that sometimes even licensed professionals (such as the aforementioned Christine Daniels) can let themselves be seduced into committing fraud. This is why it is important to look at more than the credentials; if one has proper credentials and yet continues to use "secret" formulas, use unproven methods, charge excessive fees, or denounce conventional methods you need to seek your treatment elsewhere regardless of credentials. Please be very careful because when it comes to cancer you do not get a "do-over" if you waste your time with the wrong practitioner.

Chapter 2
HOLISTIC OVERVIEW ON CANCER

Because cancer is so intrusive in a person's life receiving a cancer diagnosis is an alarming thing for *anyone*. You may feel frightened. You may feel a sense of loss of control. You may already dread the aggressive treatments you know you'll need before you've even begun treatment. Even the strongest minded person may feel overwhelmed by such a diagnosis. These feelings are normal, and they are valid, but these feeling do not need to take over your life. The first thing you need to do when you have been diagnosed is set up a support system to help you through this emotional upheaval. Do not be afraid to rely on family members and close friends who are willing to help you through this. If you do not have a close friend or nearby family member that you can lean on do not give up hope as there are support options still available to you. Do not be afraid to seek support from your local house of worship, community cancer support groups, online cancer support groups, social media-based support groups, support groups associated with local charities, and support groups associated with your local hospital or cancer treatment facility. You can either perform an Internet search to find these groups or ask your oncologist if he or she knows locations and times of some of the groups. You are not alone in your diagnosis and a circle of other people who are going through the same things that you are will invigorate your spirit and lighten your load. This alone is a tremendous step towards regrouping yourself and battling the disease.

The second thing you need to do is start educating yourself regarding your type of cancer. Keep in mind that "cancer' is not a single disease; each kind of cancer is its own disease separate from other cancers which is why no two cancers are treated the same. Education, however, empowers you; for the more you know what you are dealing with and how to deal with it, the bigger the advantage you have over the disease process. In short, education puts *you* in control of the disease, not the other way around. Start by directing all of your concerns and questions to your oncologist. He or she is there to help you understand, so do not feel you are wasting your doctor's time – answering your questions is an expected part of your doctor's job. You should also inquire whether your local hospital or cancer treatment facility has a library of educational cancer materials you can borrow from. If you are seeking information on the Internet be sure to use caution and do not blindly believe everything you read online. Make sure you are using reputable websites run by credible organizations such as (*italics* = holistic organizations):

- *National Center for Complementary and Integrative Health*
- *Office of Cancer Complementary and Alternative Medicine*
- The Sidney Kimmel Comprehensive Cancer Center
- Memorial Sloan Kettering Cancer Center
- American Institute for Cancer Research
- Cancer Treatment Centers of America
- *Society for Integrative Oncology*

- World Cancer Research Fund
- MD Anderson Cancer Center
- Dana-Farber Cancer Institute
- Center for Cancer Research
- American Cancer Society
- Cancer Research Institute
- National Cancer Institute
- Cancer Research UK
- *Cameoprogram.org*
- *Cam-Cancer.org*
- Cancer.net

If you decide to also look at *other* professionals, organizations or websites be sure that the given information is accurate – do they have scientifically proven references to support their statements? Do not rely on testimonials alone as these are heavily biased, and do not subscribe to those who try to convince you that conventional treatments are the devil. Although it is true that conventional treatments can be very hard on your body you need to be mindful that your fight against cancer is a war, and war is difficult even when you are on the winning side – you will not destroy the enemy by being gentle. Although holistic treatments can help strengthen your fight against cancer you will still need the more aggressive methods used in conventional medicine in order to actually destroy the cancer.

The third thing you need to do is make sure you are comfortable with your choice of oncologist. There is no offense in checking a physician's professional record and background. This is not a matter of mistrust, it is a matter of *your* health, and you deserve to make sure you have a qualified, ethical professional treating you. When you check into a physician do more than look at his or her professional profile; you should also search the physician's name on your state's medical board website. Do not be afraid to ask questions of the board if you do not feel sufficient information is listed. For a small fee you can also order a full report on your doctor from the Federation of State Medical Boards. There is one thing to keep in mind through your investigation though: Sometimes doctors do everything right, are not at fault, and yet a patient *still* does poorly – it just happens, unfortunately. As a result the patient or a family member may still sue for malpractice even though there is no actual blame on the doctor. It has been said that, on the average, doctors are sued for malpractice every seven years or so; therefore I caution you to refrain from jumping to conclusions prematurely if you see something that may be questionable. Be reasonable.

AN OUTLINE ON CANCER

In its most basic definition cancer is a disease process in which an uncontrolled growth of abnormal cells occurs. Unlike normal healthy cells, cancer cells do not die naturally and so they continue to multiply uncontrolled, thus creating more abnormal cells. As this number of cancer cells continues to increase a clump of cancerous tissue, known as a tumor, is usually formed (certain types of cancers, such as leukemias and sometimes inflammatory breast cancer, do not form tumors). Not all tumors are cancerous, therefore if a tumor is detected your doctor should order a biopsy[7] of the tissue to test for the presence of cancer.

In healthy cells all of the cells of the same tissue bind together and remain in their designated locations. If they become separated from their assigned locations they die through a process of self-destruction called apoptosis (pronounced *ă-POP-toe-sis*). Cancer cells are different: Their self-destruct mechanisms no longer function, therefore when a cancer cell forms it remains alive and multiplies whether it stays put or becomes separated from its group. Just how does a normal, healthy cell become a cancer cell in the first place? First, it is important to realize that all of your body cells are very active even though you do not feel it. They are constantly receiving signals from their own inner parts as well as from the other cells which surround them. Let's start with a healthy, normal cell and follow it through the changes:

The cell starts off normal and usual, performing all the tasks and functions that it is supposed to do. It responds to the signals it receives, and when it receives enough "grow" signals it responds by getting ready to multiply by way of mitosis (pronounced *my-TOE-sis*). Mitosis is a non-sexual method of reproduction in which the cell replicates its own genetic material (DNA)[8] to create a clone of itself. Once cloned, the original cell *and* the clone are both referred to as "daughter cells." Once a cell has multiplied itself a certain number of times it will normally die by apoptosis and is replaced by other, newer and healthier, replicating cells. This particular cell that we're following, though, happened to make a mistake when it replicated its DNA and so now the the daughter cell has a mistake, i.e. mutation, in its genes. This mutation can be replicated during the daughter cell's next rounds of mitosis thus creating more daughter cells with the same mutation. But your body has a way to help prevent mutations from spreading: A special gene is contained within your cells, known as p53. Its job is to look for mutations and activate other genes to repair them. If the damage is too severe to repair then p53 orders the cell to self-destruct (apoptosis) thus eliminating the problem. At least, that what *usually* happens. In the case of our mutant daughter cell here the mutation is located within the p53 gene itself; with a now-crippled p53 gene other new mutations may also arise from one generation of the mutant daughter cells to the next in that cell line. When a mutation finally occurs which eliminates the self-destruct signals in a cell, that cell becomes immortal,[9] and begins to multiply abnormally, it is now a cancer. If left alone, this cancer begins to grow through the process of angiogenesis (pronounced *AN-jee-oh-JEN-ih-sis)* described under the next subheading.

So now the question is: What happened to cause these mutations in the first place? There is no single answer as there are many causes of genetic mutations:

---

7   Biopsy: Taking a small sample of affected tissue to examine whether it is cancerous.

8   DNA = <u>D</u>eoxyribo<u>n</u>ucleic <u>A</u>cid, the building block of genes. Groups of genes are known as chromosomes.

9   Immortality of cancer cells is no exaggeration. Biomedical researchers today are still performing studies using the HeLa cervical cancer cell line which was originally harvested from a patient in 1951.

Heredity, chemical exposure, radiation exposure, food additives and preservatives, environmental poisons, high fat diets, tobacco use, excessive exposure to UV light,[10] over-consumption of alcohol, pollution, and chronic inflammation are many of the known factors for the development of different cancers. Substances known to cause cancer are called carcinogenic ("*carcino*"= cancer, "*genic*"= forming).

ANGIOGENESIS & METASTASIS

Angiogenesis is the creation of new blood vessels ("*angio*" = blood vessel, "*genesis*" = formation). Usually, angiogenesis is a good thing because without it babies could not form in the womb, surgery patients could not heal from their procedures, and accident victims could not heal from their wounds. Normal body cells have checks and balances to know when to "turn on" and "turn off" the angiogenic process. However, when it comes to cancerous cells angiogenesis is the beginning of something very very wrong. Let me explain:

It is a known fact that all healthy body cells need an aerobic environment, i.e. oxygen, in order to grow and thrive. These cells obtain their supply of oxygen via the circulatory system – the blood vessels. Now, sometimes it is touted by some holistic practitioners that cancer cells are the opposite; they need an *anaerobic* environment, i.e. low-oxygen setting, in order to thrive. They base this on a theory originated from Nobel prize recipient Dr. Otto Warburg, M.D. which was published in the 1930's. Dr. Warburg noted that cancer cells have a lower respiration rate than healthy cells, thus he theorized that cancer cells would die when exposed to greater concentrations of oxygen. This gave rise to the oxygen-based cancer therapies we see in some holistic practices today. Later, however, Dr. Warburg's theory was shown to be in error: In 1971 Dr. Moses Judah Folkman discovered that cancer tumors are actually dependent on angiogenesis – the formation of blood vessels – in order to thrive.[11] Research based on Dr. Folkman's discoveries has shown that cancer tumors do, indeed, create their own network of blood vessels and will only thrive if these blood vessels are allowed to remain. A tumor's vessels are always connected directly to the body's regular circulatory system, thus the growing tumor is receiving the same level of oxygenation as the healthy cells, ergo it is *thriving in an oxygenated* environment. As a matter of fact, cancer treatments which block the process of angiogenesis in tumors (thus cutting off their oxygen supply) is one of the most effective methods in destroying tumors. Although Dr. Warburg was a brilliant doctor and scientist, he was clearly wrong on this one particular theory.[12]

When a tumor is very small it can get by on the oxygen available from the nearby blood vessels immediately surrounding it. However, as it grows, its need for oxygen likewise grows. Without its *own* blood supply the tumor will not be able to grow very large, will weaken, and will die. For its own survival the tiny tumor must prompt surrounding blood vessels to begin creating new vessel pathways directly into

---

10 UV = Ultraviolet, a form of radiation which induces tanning in your skin. Overexposure usually happens due to excessive time spent tanning in the sunlight or in tanning beds.

11 *Tumor Angiogenesis: Therapeutic Implications*" (Folkman, M.D. 1971)

12 Although science has shown that cancerous cells *do* have a lowered respiration rate than healthy cells,this does not lower the cells' need for oxygen.

the tumor itself. The tumor usually does this through the use of **V**ascular **E**ndothelial **G**rowth **F**actor, a.k.a. VEGF, a protein formed by cancers which promotes angiogenesis. Once these already-existing blood vessels hook up their "piping" into the tumor, the tumor is able to continue its growth, *AND*, because the tumor is now directly hooked up to the circulatory system, if some of the cancer cells happen to break off from the now-enlarging tumor they can wash into the connected blood vessel system, land somewhere else in the body, and begin a new tumor at the new landing site. In other words, if a breast cancer cell breaks off your breast tumor and washes downstream via your blood vessels and lands on your liver you will begin to grow a breast cancer tumor on your liver. Although it is on your liver the cells are still mutated breast cells; therefore this is not liver cancer, it is still breast cancer, just no longer in the breast. As this new breast cancer tumor grows on your liver and produces a new blood vessel system for itself another cell may break off from *this* tumor and be carried to your brain. Now you have a breast cancer tumor in your breast, on your liver *and* on your brain. This process of spreading is known as metastasis. Because all these new tumors are still breast cancer cells, regardless of where they are growing, they will only respond to treatment for breast cancer; therefore you will continue to receive treatment for breast cancer, not liver or brain cancer.

Your circulatory system is not the only way for metastasis to occur, as sometimes cancer cells will, instead, wash into your lymph (pronounced "*limf*") system. Since your lymph system circulates other fluids throughout your body this can also be a pathway for cancer cells to circulate. If a cancer cell rides the lymph system it can land in a lymph node – a filtration station of sorts – and start growing a tumor there. This is a common situation which is often why some cancer patients must have lymph nodes removed during treatment.

When a person is discovered to have cancer the oncologist will "stage" the disease to see how far it has progressed. The stage of progression helps dictate the treatment plan to be chosen for the patient. Here is a list of the stages and what they mean:

Stage	What It Means[13]
Stage 0	At this stage the tumor is tiny and non-invasive. It is oftentimes referred to as a "carcinoma in situ" and is sometimes interpreted as a "pre-cancerous condition." With prompt treatment the patient has a 100% survival rate.
Stage 1	The tumor has grown and is just beginning to invade surrounding tissues. At this point your cancer is considered to be "localized." Though it takes a little more effort, it is still one of the easier stages to treat. Prompt treatment gives patients up to a 100% survival rate. (Some sources cite 98%).
Stage 2	Now the tumor is growing more deeply into neighboring tissues and nearby lymph nodes. The patient may start experiencing mild or

13 Survival rates are based on a five year period after finishing treatment.

Stage	What It Means
	vague symptoms depending on where the tumor is located. Prompt treatment gives patients up to a 93% survival rate.
Stage 3	At this point the tumor is growing large enough to spread to other lymph nodes and muscles. At this stage it is tougher to treat, but not impossible to win. With prompt treatment patients have up to a 72% survival rate – which is still very good.
Stage 4	This is the last stage. The various tumors growing in the nearby lymph nodes and muscles grow large enough so that pieces of the tumors break off and circulate in the body via the lymph or circulatory systems. These pieces attach to distant organs and lymph nodes and begin making new tumors at these locations, such as your liver, intestines, brain, or elsewhere. This is the most difficult stage to treat, but still not impossible to survive. With aggressive treatment patients have up to a 22% survival rate – although this may seem daunting, it is still not an impossible fight.

Clearly, the earlier you discover the cancer the better your chances. This is why it is so important for people to schedule all of their cancer screening tests on a regular basis. When you have already been diagnosed with a cancer it is equally important to keep up with all of your treatments and continue scheduling your post-cancer check-ups on a regular basis after your treatments have been completed. And, if you happen to be diagnosed with a late-stage cancer do not let that diagnosis scare you: There are innumerable cancer patients "living with mets" (living with metastasis) who have managed to live with it as a chronic condition for ten years or more, continuing to live nearly-normal lives day by day while maintaining treatment.

YOUR IMMUNE SYSTEM

The function of your immune system is an extremely important element in your fight against cancer. Let me explain: In normal circumstances your immune system is an army of specialized cells which hunt down and destroy foreign invaders in your body. In your immune system's point of view, any organism in the body that is not "self" is a foreign invader and must be destroyed: The immune response is triggered by the presence of certain proteins that are given off by the invaders; proteins which scream *"Not Self!"* to the immune system. When the immune system receives this signal it immediately activates and send out its army of fighters to seek and destroy. This is what happens when your immune system detects dangerous bacteria, fungi, viruses, molds, and parasites. Even patients receiving organ transplants are at lifetime risk of a major immune response against the transplanted organ (because it is of someone else's "self" and not your own) requiring them to remain on immune suppressing medications for the rest of their lives.

Even though cancer cells have a changed DNA (due to the mutations), you need to remember that they originated from your own normal body cells. As such, in the beginning of their mutations they do not look very different from normal body cells to your immune system, and so they continue to multiply undetected at first. Over time, though, as the cancer cells continue their mutations they may begin to emit certain proteins which are no longer the normal "self", triggering an immune response. The immune system then sends specialized proteins known as cytokines and cells known as Natural Killer cells (NK)[14] to eradicate the cancerous offenders. Oftentimes your NK cells will respond fast enough to destroy the mutant cells before a cancer can fully develop and you are none the wiser.

In many cases though, the cancer cells are able to slip past the immune system by either (a) developing mutations that allow them to avoid detection by the immune system, or (b) taking a while to emit the mutant proteins which trigger the immune response. And, if you happen to develop an especially fast growing type of cancer, the cancer cells may multiply too quickly for your immune system to keep up once it is finally triggered. It is these circumstances which allows cancer to take a foothold.

CACHEXIA

Cachexia (pronounced: Ka-KEX-ee-uh) is a condition in which a chronically ill patient starts to lose body fat and muscle; it is a complication commonly seen in advanced stages of HIV, tuberculosis, cancers, and other chronic diseases. It is not caused by lack of calories but instead is caused by a changed metabolism resulting from the illness itself; in this case, cancer. A normal metabolism is primarily anabolic, meaning it allows for cell growth and regular maintenance. Cachexia, however, is the result of a metabolism which has turned *catabolic* – one that promotes cell destruction. This is why cachexia is very debilitating, decreases quality of life and severely limits the continuation of cancer treatments. If cachexia is not reversed a cancer patient's quality of life and survival rate is significantly reduced. Yes, this does sound scary, but medical science gives a lot of hope. Let me briefly explain how cachexia starts and what can be done about it:

Although it is not yet *fully* understood how the mechanisms behind the onset of cachexia work, scientists believe it may be initiated by inflammation induced by cytokines.[15] This is how it works: When a bacteria, virus, parasite, mold, or tumor is detected by the immune system (your white blood cells) your immune system releases cytokines – "messenger" molecules whose job is to call more white blood cells to come and help attack the problem. This causes an inflammatory response in your body. When an *excessive* amount of inflammatory cytokines are released over a long period of time it causes negative effects in the body.[16] For example, some

---

14   Natural killer cells are a type of white blood cell capable of binding to tumor cells and injecting them with perforin, a protein which punches holes in the tumor cell walls, thus killing them.

15   *Effects of anti-parathyroid hormone-related protein monoclonal antibody and osteoprotegerin on PTHrP-producing tumor-induced cachexia in nude mice* (Haruo Iguchi, 2006); *Systemic inflammation, cachexia and prognosis in patients with cancer* (C. Deans, 2005); *Cytokines and cachexia* (P. Matthys, 1997)

16   Cytokines commonly associated with cachexia include Tumor Necrosis Factor (TNF), interleukin-6, gamma interferon, myokines, and a substance secreted from cancer tumors known as proteolysis-inducing factor.

cytokines activate substances which reduce muscle protein synthesis, while others initiate catabolysis – the breakdown of skeletal muscle tissue.[17] Other cytokines seem to change a patient's fatty tissue from white fat (which stores calories) to brown fat (which burns calories), thus tapping out your body's energy reserves.

Another element which may contribute to the development of cachexia is thought to be a protein released by the cancer tumor itself, a protein known as Parathyroid Hormone-related Protein (PTHrP). Research has shown that this substance may cause metabolic changes in your fatty tissues in ways that promote energy burning instead of energy storage.[18] One study exploring the action of PTHrP in cachexic patients with lung and colon cancer found that, out of the 47 patients being studied, 17 of them (36%) were found to have elevated levels of PTHrP in their blood samples; these same 17 patients were also shown to be producing more heat energy during rest than the remaining ones in the group of patients.[19]

Yet another possible contributor to cachexia is the process in which cancer cells create the energy they live on. Normal cells manufacture their own energy by processing oxygen and glucose through their specialized "power-station" organs, known as mitochondria (MY-toe-KONN-dree-uh). Cancer cells, on the other hand, manufacture their energy by fermenting glucose. This is how it works: Cancer cells ferment the glucose, causing them to excrete a waste product known as *lactic acid*, which is not useful to the body. The body rids itself of the lactic acid by breaking it down in the liver, resulting in by-products such as glucose. This glucose is then circulated back to the tumor and fermented by the cancer cells to create more energy for themselves. This burning of glucose by the cancer cells results in the creation of more lactic acid which, again, results in more glucose after the liver breaks it down. This cycle of glucose and lactic acid is known in oncology as "*The Warburg Effect*", named for Dr. Otto Warburg who discovered this cycle. Because a cancer cell's ability to manufacture energy from glucose is much less efficient than a normal cell's mitochondrial process the tumor requires a large amount of glucose to thrive. As a result, the body's supply of glucose quickly becomes depleted, requiring the body to manufacture more glucose, known as gluconeogenesis (*gluco* = sugar, *neo* = new, *genesis* = formation) in order to take care of its other functions. If enough glucose is not consumed by the patients, the only way the body can build up more glucose is by breaking down fatty acids and muscle tissues in order to create the necessary amounts of glucose needed. This results in the characteristic weight loss and gaunt appearance common to people with cachexia. In order to reverse cachexia this cycle of catabolic metabolism must be broken.

Even though a cachexic patient will look under-nourished, the mechanisms of cachexia are complex and cannot be reversed simply by feeding the patient nutritious food. Because cachexia is brought on by a number of metabolic changes scientists are

---

17 Skeletal muscles are the ones directly attached to your bones. This is in contrast to other muscles located within your organs.

18 *Tumor-derived PTH-related protein triggers adipose tissue browning and cancer cachexia* (Serkan Kir, 2014)

19 **Harvard Gazette**, July 13, 2014, "*Antibody Halts Cancer-Related Wasting Condition*" Richard Saltus, Dana-Farber Cancer Institute Communications

challenged to find a cure that works across the board; thus they work tirelessly exploring new ways to reverse this condition. This has resulted in some encouraging finds such as:

- *Anti-PTHrP Antibodies*: In vivo studies have shown that applying a combination of osteoprotegerin with anti-PTHrP antibodies can neutralize PTHrP and significantly decrease cachexia in laboratory mice.[20]

- *Glucogenic blockers*: These are prescription medications that may block the production of glucose in the liver. One particular diabetic medication, Metformin, is being studied for its use in reversing cachexia.[21]

- *Hydrazine Sulfate:* This is a supplement that is thought to block the production of glucose in the liver. This is discussed in detail in chapter 11 of this book.

- *Ketogenic Diet:* This is a specialized diet thought to inhibit the production of glucose by significantly decreasing the patient's intake of carbohydrates. This is discussed in detail in chapter 8 of this book.

- *Myostatin Blocks*: In a study using mouse models it was found that overproduction of muscle-inhibiting proteins known as myostatins can also be key in the onset of cachexia, and that blocking the cell receptors for myostatin can successfully reverse the process of cachexia, prolonging survival.[22]

- *NSAIDS*: a.k.a. Non-steroidal Anti-inflammatory Drugs; these work by reducing inflammation-causing substances. Commonly known over-the-counter NSAIDS include aspirin, acetaminophen (Tylenol) and Ibuprofen (Advil). Although several clinical trials have shown that use of these medications show positive results in patient weight gain, quality of life, and survival, more study documentation needs to be completed before using NSAIDS as a broad treatment for cachexia.[23] One particular NSAID known as Indomethacin has been shown in clinical trials to double the survival rate of cachexic patients.[24]

---

20 *Effects of anti-parathyroid hormone-related protein monoclonal antibody and osteoprotegerin on PTHrP-producing tumor-induced cachexia in nude mice* (Haruo Iguchi, 2006)
21 *Cancer cachexia and diabetes: similarities in metabolic alterations and possible treatment* (S. Chevalier, 2014)
22 *Reversal of Cancer Cachexia and Muscle Wasting by ActRIIB Antagonism Leads to Prolonged Survival* (Xiaolan Zhou, 2010)
23 *Non-steroidal anti-inflammatory drugs for the treatment of cancer cachexia: a systematic review* (J Reid, 2013)
24 *Anti-inflammatory treatment may prolong survival in undernourished patients with metastatic solid tumors* (K. Lundholm, 1994)

- *Glutamine cocktail*: Studies have shown that combining glutamine with with beta–hydroxy-beta-methylbutyrate (HMB) and arginine can help reduce cachexia

If you are looking for natural alternatives instead there are some plant-based items that may help control cachexia via inhibition of inflammation. Discuss these with your prescribing physicians and holistic practitioners before using (See chapter 6 of this book for details on the following herbs and supplements).

HERB	IMPORTANT INFORMATION
Boswellia *Boswellia Serrata*	Also known as Indian Frankincense. This is a powerful anti-inflammatory herb due to the presence of boswellic acids. Do not confuse this with frankincense made from Norwegian fir trees or myrrh.
Bu Zhong Yi Qi Chinese formula	Also known as Hochuekkito in Japanese medicine, animal studies have shown this formula to alleviate cachexia.
Cat's Claw *Uncaria Tomentosa (or)* *Uncaria guianensis*	Studies have shown that cat's claw inhibits production of Tumor Necrosis Factor, (TNF), a cytokine which, when produced over a length of time, may contribute to cachexia.
Cloves *Eugenia Caryophyllata* *or* *Syzygium aromaticum*	Studies have shown that eugenol, a substance in cloves, can inhibit the production of interleukins, a family of cytokines known to contribute to cachexia.[25]
Devil's Claw *Harpagophytum* *procumbens*	This south African plant contains iridoid glycosides, especially one called harpagoside, which reduces inflammation. In vivo studies show that devil's claw can inhibit the production of certain interleukins and TNF, cytokines known to contribute to cachexia.
Ginger *Zingiber officinale*	Ginger contains gingerols and zerumbone. In vivo studies have shown these to inhibit the production of cytokines that are known to contribute to cachexia.
Guarana *Paullinia cupana*	This tropical herb has been shown to stabilize weight loss and increase appetite in patients with advanced cancers.
Hydroxymethyl-butyrate	Also known as HMB, this substance is created by your own body when metabolizing an amino acid known as leucine, therefore intake of leucine in your diet can be important.
Omega 3's[26]	Clinical trials were performed using omega 3 fatty acids from

---

25 Clove and eugenol in noncytotoxic concentrations exert immunomodulatory/anti-inflammatory action on cytokine production by murine macrophages (Bachiega, 2012)

26 Fish oils have the omega 3 fatty acids known as eicosapentaenoic acid (EPA) and docosahexaenoic acid (DHA). Plant oils have the omega 3's known as alpha-linolenic acids (ALA).

HERB	IMPORTANT INFORMATION
	fish oils which showed that intake of these Omega 3's may reduce cachexia if patients begin taking it during the very early stages of condition. There is also some evidence that omega 3's can preserve muscle mass even when taken during a course of chemotherapy treatment.
Rosemary *Rosmarinus officinalis*	In a review of studies it was shown that Rosemary contains many substances which can inhibit inflammatory cytokines as well as induce apoptosis in cancer cells.

Although cachexia can be induced by a prolonged cytokine response keep aware that you do need *some* cytokines to help destroy your cancer. If you have *not* developed cachexia then do not be afraid to discuss immune-stimulating agents such as elderberry or shiitake mushrooms with your oncologist or holistic practitioner. If you choose to use immune-stimulating supplements be sure that you do not exceed dosages recommended by your physician or holistic practitioners because over-stimulation of your immune system may induce cachexia. Do not use more than one immune-stimulant at a time unless your physician advises otherwise. Moderation is key. If during your course of cancer treatment you do develop cachexia I strongly recommend you discontinue using supplements which stimulate the immune system.

Chapter 3
CHEMOTHERAPY DRUG CLASSES

Because there are hundreds of different types of cancer there are also hundreds of different chemotherapy agents currently in use in the fight against cancer; these agents are grouped into categories, i.e. classes. Each class of chemotherapy drugs is specific to the way in which it fights cancer. It is important to know which class your prescribed agents are categorized under as this makes a difference in what to expect in regards to side effects and possible health risks. Speak to your oncologist if you are unsure which class your chemotherapy agent(s) fall under or if you have any questions regarding your prescribed agents.

ALKYLATING AGENTS

Alkylating agents are the most commonly used chemotherapy drugs, and although they can be used for many kinds of cancers they tend to work better on slower growing tumors. Alkylating agents work by binding directly to the cancer cells' DNA strands in several places resulting in mutations which cause them to be unable to multiply (either by cell death or inability to reproduce). When enough cancer cells are deactivated with these agents the tumor is destroyed. Although this damage to DNA is necessary to destroy the cancer, it does carry the risk of potential damage to bone marrow.[27] In rare cases this may lead to the development of acute myelogenous leukemia (AML) within ten years after treatment is finished. Fortunately, this risk is "dose-dependent," which means lower doses of these agents result in a lower risk. I strongly encourage you to speak with your oncologist if you have concerns about this risk.

Alkylating agents are further categorized into sub-classes: Alkyl sulfonates, ethylenimines, hydrazines, nitrogen mustards, nitrosureas, and triazines. Nitrosureas have the ability to cross the blood-brain barrier making them an effective treatment for patients diagnosed with brain tumors. The blood-brain barrier is filtering system built into the brain and spinal cord to keep certain types of harmful molecules out of the central nervous system.

The biggest hurdle with alkylating agents is that sometimes the cancer cells can develop a resistance to them, rendering the drugs less effective against the cancer. This sometimes happens because the cancer cells make use of a certain enzyme, MGMT,[28] that is designed to repair DNA damage. In normal, healthy cells this enzyme is crucial, but in cancer cells this can become a problem as you do not want them repairing themselves. Fortunately, there are prescription drugs as well as holistic methods which can be added to your treatment plan to inhibit this enzyme and reduce

---

27 Bone marrow: Soft tissue in the center of bones. In adults the flat bones (hips, ribs, skull, shoulder blades) contain red marrow which creates blood components. Certain bone marrow problems may cause the development of leukemias, also known as blood cancers.

28 (A.k.a. Omega 6-Methylguanine DNA methyltransferase.) *O6-methylguanine DNA methyltransferase as a promising target for the treatment of temozolomide-resistant gliomas.* (Fan, 2013)

22

the chemo-resistance. Some well-known alkylating agents include: Busulfan, cyclophosphamide, carmustine, dacarbazine, temozolomide and thiotepa.

ANTIMETABOLITES

Because antimetabolite agents are so similar to some of your body's own natural substances an agent can interfere with cancer cell growth by substituting itself for some of the genetic material being built during cancer cell reproduction. This can result in either cancer cell death or simply render the cancer cell unable to multiply depending upon the agent used and the type of cancer being targeted. Sub-classes of antimetabolites include folic acid analogues, pyrimidine analogues, and purine analogues.

Pyrimidine analogues, a.k.a. pyrimidine antagonists, tend to be associated with a risk for liver and gall bladder injury, therefore you should be sure your oncologist knows if you have any past or present problems with your liver or gall bladder. In most cases these risks are related to dosage and method of delivery, depending upon the particular agent being used.

Purine analogues, a.k.a. purine antagonists, tend to be associated with an increased risk in developing infections. There is only a handful of purine analogues that are relevant for cancer treatment. Studies have shown that the application of resveratrol along with purine analogues when treating for chronic lymphocytic leukemia (CLL) helped increase cancer cell self-destruction without harming surrounding healthy cells. According to one study *"[resveratrol] may be used as a single agent, especially in older persons for whom there are some limitations for the use of aggressive treatment...a lower purine analogue dose could potentially be used in combination with resveratrol because of their combined effect."*[29]

Folate analogues, a.k.a. folate antagonists, are substances which decrease the production of folic acid, also known as vitamin B9. Folic acid is essential for the formation of nucleotides which are the basic building blocks of DNA. Research has found that leukemia patients whose diets were low in folate / folic acid also had lower white blood cell counts than leukemia patients who had normal levels of folate in their diets. This observation eventually led to the development of the folate antagonist methotrexate, which is one of the most commonly used folate antagonists today as it is effective against several types of cancers. One big drawback to methotrexate treatment is that drug resistance is a common issue.

ANTITUMOR ANTIBIOTICS

Anti-tumor antibiotics, a.k.a. anti-neoplastic antibiotics, are produced from a bacteria species known as *Streptomyces* which was found to have anti-tumor properties in the 1960's.[30] These types of antibiotics are not like antibiotics made for treating infections, instead these antibiotics work against cancer cells by changing the DNA inside them thus preventing them from multiplying. This class of agents is

---

29 *Resveratrol Increases Rate of Apoptosis Caused by Purine Analogues in Malignant Lymphocytes of Chronic Lymphocytic Leukemia* (Podhorecka, 2011)

30 Streptomyces is a spore-producing bacteria which resembles a fungus, therefore some sources erroneously identify this microorganism as a fungus.

divided into three sub-classes: anthracyclines, chromomycins, and miscellaneous.

Anthracyclines are known to increase survival rates but are also a known risk in causing irreversible heart damage, especially in the left ventricle of the heart.[31] Due to this risk there are oftentimes lifetime dose limitations put in place to protect the organ. This means individual patients are not allowed to continue treatment with anthracyclines once they've reach a certain level of exposure to them. A study published in 2014 showed that a high intake of iron during anthracycline treatment tended to increase the risk of heart damage in patients using anthracyclines,[32] therefore your iron levels should be monitored during treatment. Do not take iron supplements or eat a diet high in iron-rich foods without discussing this with your oncologist first.[33] Because of the risk of heart damage patients using this class of agents are carefully monitored to ensure heart health. Anthracyclines include: Daunorubicin, doxorubicin, epirubicin,[34] idarubicin, mitoxantrone, and valrubicin. Anthracyclines are also known as topoisomerase II inhibitors, which carries a low risk of developing mixed lineage leukemia (MLL) after treatment is complete. Fortunately, leukemias caused from topoisomerase II inhibitors are of the easier types to treat.

Chromomycins include Actinomycin-D (a.k.a. dactinomycin)[35] oligomycin, olivomycin, mithramycin, and plicamycin. At the turn of the millennium plicamycin and mithramycin were withdrawn from the market due to their extremely toxic properties.

Miscellaneous agents include bleomycin and mitomycin. Bleomycin's most notorious side effect is scarring of the lungs (a.k.a. pulmonary fibrosis), therefore if you already have breathing issues or other health issues with your lungs you must be sure your oncologist is aware before you take bleomycin. This scarring is more likely to occur in elderly patients and those who have been given a higher total dose of the agent. In contrast, mitomycin's effects on the lungs is much rarer.

In general, anti-tumor antibiotics are known for also causing bone marrow suppression, liver problems, and kidney problems. Be sure you speak with your oncologist about the risks involved and what it means for your health before using these agents.

CORTICOSTEROIDS

Corticosteroids are a steroid-based substance naturally made in your adrenal glands (which sit atop each kidney). When a patient is given prescription corticosteroids the adrenal glands tend to reduce their production of the substance.

---

31 The heart has four chambers for blood flow: Two upper chambers called the atria, and two lower chambers called the ventricles.

32 *The role of iron in anthracycline cardiotoxicity* (Elena Gammella, 2014)

33 Foods high in iron include: Red meats, pork, poultry, seafood, beans, dark greens leafy vegetables, dried fruits, and fortified cereals. Iron from animal-based foods is more easily absorbed in your body than iron from plant foods. Vitamin C products and supplements also increase absorption of iron.

34 Epirubicin is less damaging to the heart than doxorubicin, though a risk does remain.

35 Actinomycin-D is also known as a polypeptide antibiotic.

Therefore, when you no longer need the prescription you will need to slowly wean yourself off the drugs to give your adrenal glands a chance to begin increasing production again. The most common forms of corticosteroids prescribed are dexamethasone, hydrocortisone, methylprednisolone, prednisolone, and prednisone. Because corticosteroids affect the adrenal glands most patients are not ordered to have long-term corticosteroid treatment. Never suddenly stop taking your corticosteroids without your prescribing physician's oversight. The length of your corticosteroid treatment depends upon the type of cancer you have and which other treatment(s) you are being prescribed.

Corticosteroids have many uses when it comes to treating cancer, including the reduction of inflammation, reduction in the immune response after a bone marrow transplant, increase in appetite, and reduction of some of the side effects caused by certain chemotherapy regimens. Corticosteroids can be given as an oral medication, an intramuscular injection, or as an injection into your vein.

Side effects of corticosteroid treatment may include: Digestive problems, insomnia, yeast infection, anxiety, weight gain, cataracts, osteoporosis, thinning of the skin, increased risk of infection, and slower wound healing. Other side effects may occur; speak to your prescribing physician.

Precautions: Because corticosteroids inhibit the immune system patients using them must avoid people who have an active infection with chicken pox or shingles. They should also avoid any live vaccinations.

DIFFERANTIATING AGENTS

Differentiating therapy is founded on the idea that certain types of cancer cells were normal cells which were stunted or have reverted to an immature state resulting in a lack of their ability to control their growth. Differentiation therapy is used to "reboot" the cancer cell to re-start the process of maturation in order to return to a normal state and regain control of their growth. Instead of destroying the cells this form of therapy reigns in their growth to allow conventional chemotherapy agents to destroy the cancerous cells. Because differentiating agents are not actually killing any cells they tend to be less toxic and cause less side effects than other chemotherapy agents.

Differentiating agents tend to be retinoid-based substances which are similar to vitamin A. The first differentiating agent to be discovered was Tretinoin,[36] a topical acne treatment, which has been shown to also induce complete remission in roughly 70% of acute promyelocytic leukemia (APL) cases when used as an oral agent. Patients should not take this to mean they should orally consume their prescription acne treatments for their leukemia, as acne treatments are not formulated for oral consumption. Leukemia patients using this agent are usually patients who do not respond to, or cannot use, anthracycline agents. It is not used as maintenance therapy in such patients. When used for leukemia there may be side effects such as blood clots, liver damage, bleeding disorders, pneumonia, digestive issues, weight changes, heart problems, blood pressure issues, and pain. Although differentiating agents are

---

36 Also known as all-trans-retinoic acid (ATRA).

commonly used for different types of leukemia researchers are also looking into the potential for using them against solid tumors as well.

EPOTHILONES

Epothilones are anti-tumor substances derived from a bacteria known as *Sorangium cellulosum*. There are several known epothilones identified as Epothilones A -F, which have been tested in laboratories and in human cancer patients. Epothilones are known as mitotic inhibitors[37] and perform similar to the action of taxanes (see the subheading "Plant Alkaloids" in this chapter). Although similar to taxanes the epothilones, unlike taxanes, tend to be more readily dissolved in water whereas taxanes need solvents to allow the taxanes to mix with water. These solvents may cause toxic effects on a patient's heart, therefore epothilones may be preferred for patients with certain health issues. Research has also observed that Epothilone-B does not induce the inflammatory response common to taxanes such as paclitaxel. In most cases epothilones are combined with other chemotherapy agents to better target the specific cancer being treated. Usually the combination is administered as an intravenous treatment.

Although epothilones have benefits over taxanes these are not without side effects. The most common side effects tend to be weakness and pain in the joints. Less common side effects include mouth sores and headaches.

IMMUNOTHERAPY

Cancer immunotherapy, also known as biologic therapy, is a system of treatment in which a patient's immune system is used to help fight the cancer. This can be accomplished in two ways: (1) Stimulating the patient's own immune system to work harder against the cancer, or (2) Giving immune system components to the patient from an outside source. Immunotherapy works better on some types of cancer than it does on others. Immunotherapy can come in various forms such as: Targeted therapy (monoclonal antibodies), cancer vaccines including dendritic cell therapy,[38] cytokines, immune modulators, oncolytic viruses, and more.

Although immunotherapy can be a very effective treatment there are certain barriers that sometimes happen. For example, your cancer cells may not be different enough from your normal cells resulting in your immune system being unable to recognize them as dangerous. In other cases, some cancer cells may release substances which suppress the activity in your immune system. In yet other cases your immune system may simply be not strong enough to destroy the cancer.

Although this type of therapy uses biological substances it can still cause certain side effects. The side effects most commonly associated with immunotherapy include: Pain, fatigue, fever, chills, dizziness, blood pressure changes, and nausea,

---

37 "Mitotic inhibitor" means it inhibits the process of mitosis, i.e. cell replication. Also known as microtubule inhibitors or anti-microtubule agents.

38 Dendritic cell therapy was approved by the FDA in 2010. Dendritic cells are immune system components in the blood; they are not present in large amounts. Dendritic cell therapy consists of harvesting cells from the patient's blood and processing them in a laboratory to create even more dendritic cells, which are then reintroduced into the patient's blood stream en masse.

among others. Discuss with your oncologist which specific side effects you need to be aware of as different agents may produce different side effects. Immunotherapeutic agents can be administered intravenously, orally, topically, and intravesically (into your urinary bladder).

PLANT ALKALOIDS

Plant alkaloids are cell-cycle specific agents created from certain types of plants. Sub-classes of plant alkaloids include camptothecin analogs, vinca alkaloids, taxanes, and epipodophyllotoxins.

Vinca alkaloids and *taxanes* are both sub-classed as microtubule inhibitors. The vinca alkaloids are made from the periwinkle plant (*Catharanthus rosea*) and are given as an intravenous treatment. A well-known side effect of vinca alkaloids is their risk of causing neuropathy (nerve damage). As for taxanes, these agents are made from the bark of the Pacific Yew tree (*Taxus brevifolia*). A well-known side effect of taxanes is their risk of lowering blood counts in patients.

Camptothecins and *epipodophyllotoxins* are known as topoisomerase inhibitors. These inhibit the function of enzymes known as topoisomerases (enzymes involved in DNA replication) which interferes with the cancer cells' DNA structure, causing apoptosis (cancer cell suicide). Topoisomerase inhibitors are sub-classed into type I and type II, according to which enzyme they influence.[39] Camptothecin analogs are derived from the Asian *Camptotheca acuminata* tree and are classified as topoisomerase type I inhibitors. Epipodophyllotoxins are derived from the May apple tree and are classified as topoisomerase type II inhibitors. Type II inhibitors carry the low risk of developing acute myelogenous leukemia (AML).

PLATINUMS

Platinum agents are identified with the suffix "-*platin*" such as carbo<u>platin</u>, cis<u>platin</u>, and oxali<u>platin</u>. Although platinums are not alkylating agents they are oftentimes placed in that category because they perform actions similar to alkylating agents. Although platinums are less likely to cause leukemia than alkylating agents, these still carry some risk, primarily with cisplatin and carboplatin. The risk of leukemia is dose dependent; the higher the dose of the agent the higher the risk of leukemia; the risk is increased if radiation is given along with the platinum agent. A Chinese study investigated the effects of combining platinum therapy with xiaoji decoction, a TCM[40] formula. This randomized, single-blind study followed 40 patients with non-small cell lung cancer.[41] Twenty of the patients were given conventional treatment and twenty were treated with a combination of platinum agents, infusions of cytokine-induced killer cells, and the xiaoji decoction.[42] Those

---

39 Mitoxantrone, an anti-tumor antibiotic, is also sub-classed as a topoisomerase II inhibitor.
40 TCM = <u>T</u>raditional <u>C</u>hinese <u>M</u>edicine.
41 *Effect of Chinese Medicine Xiaoji Decoction Combined with Platinum-based Chemotherapy and Transfusion of Cytokine-induced Killer Cells in Patients with Stage III B/IV Non-small Cell Lung Cancer* (Li Liuning, 2015)
42 Xiaoji decoction ingredients include: Milk vetch (*Astragalus mongholicus*), turkey tail mushroom (*Coriolus versicolor*), babchi seed (*Psoralea corylifolia L*), snake needle grass (*Hedyotis diffusa*),

who were given the infusions and decoction during treatment experienced increased survival rates and longer periods of progression-free survival.[43]

Platinum-based agents may cause magnesium deficiencies in patients, therefore it is essential that you take any magnesium supplements that may be prescribed by your oncologist. Take note that too much magnesium can cause severe diarrhea and stomach cramping, heart rhythm issues, low blood pressure, confusion, and death, therefore take only the amount prescribed for you. Also, be aware that magnesium can interact with antibiotics, diuretics, blood thinners, muscle relaxers, and blood pressure medications. Let your prescribing physicians know if you have any kidney problems before starting magnesium supplementation.

TARGETED THERAPY DRUGS

Targeted therapy is a system of treatment in which specific genes or proteins in the cancer cells are targeted for interference in order to prevent the cancer cells from multiplying. This is in contrast to other chemotherapy agents which actively kill rapidly dividing cells indiscriminately. Targeted therapy may go by other names such as "molecular targeted therapies" and "precision medicine." In most cases targeted therapy is used in tandem with chemotherapy in order for the patient to get the most benefit. There are two main types of targeted therapy: Monoclonal antibodies and small-molecule agents.

Monoclonal antibodies block receptor sites on and around cell surfaces, preventing cancer cell growth. These antibodies are too large to penetrate the surface of a cancer cell however they oftentimes help funnel chemotherapy agents into the cancer cells, in effect helping your chemotherapy agents work better. Monoclonal antibody agents are usually identified by the suffix "-*mab*", (such as Labetuzumab, Trastuzumab, Vandortuzumab vedotin, etc.). These agents are usually given through intravenous methods.

Small-molecule agents are oral agents composed of molecules small enough to enter into the cancer cells to do their work; oftentimes this means blocking the process of tumor blood vessel formation (angiogenesis). Most of these agents are identified with the suffix "-*nib*" (such as crizotinib, lapatinib, trametinib, etc.), though there are a few exceptions. Many small-molecule agents are sub-classed as tyrosine kinase inhibitors, serine and threonine kinase inhibitors, and small molecule drug conjugates.

Different cancer tumors will have different targets, therefore what works for one cancer may not work for another. For example, an oncologist may be treating one woman with HER2 positive breast cancer and another woman with ER+ breast cancer. Although both are breast cancers they are each different kinds of cancer with different kinds of receptors; therefore each would require a different plan of targeted therapy. Due to these differences among tumors it is important that your oncologist

---

curcuma kwangsiensis, scorpion, centipede and rhubarb

43 Progression-free survival, a.k.a. PFS, is the length of time during and after treatment in which a patient continues to live with the cancer but it does not become worse.

orders tests to gather information about your cancer's genetics, proteins and other features in order to prescribe the most effective targeted treatment for you.

Although using targeted therapy may seem like it should be a simple matter once the information is gathered be aware that this is not always the case. Having a specific target for the agent does not guarantee that the tumor will respond to the agent. This can happen for many reasons: Sometimes the tumor becomes resistant to the therapy – this usually occurs through genetic mutations happening within the cancer cells. Sometimes a target turns out to be not as important as the doctor originally thought. Other times the side effects from the therapy may be too much for the patient to continue treatment with.

Side effects that may occur when using targeted therapy may include: Skin issues, nail problems, issues with blood clotting, slow wound healing, high blood pressure, and eye problems. Depending upon the targeting agent used there may be other side effects also. Be sure to discuss these with your prescribing physician.

Chapter 4
HOLISTIC OVERVIEW OF CHEMOTHERAPY

THE BASICS

Simply put, chemotherapy is a method of treatment using chemicals (*"chemo"*) to destroy cancerous cells. Chemotherapy drugs may also be used for various diseases, but the ones used for treating cancer are also known as antineoplastic agents (*"anti"*=against, *"neo"*=new, *"plastic"*=formation), and cytotoxic agents (*"cyto"* = cell, *"toxic"*= poison). I am not going to sugar-coat this: Because cancer is such an aggressive disease chemotherapy agents are known to be aggressive treatments; therefore they have the potential to be highly toxic. Many holistic practitioners will tell you that chemotherapy is pure poison, and in truth, it really is if it is not given correctly. Therefore, chemotherapy needs to be administered in carefully controlled doses by licensed professionals as the aim is to give patients enough of the agent to kill the cancer without harming the patients themselves. Because chemotherapy agents are so strong it is extremely important that you take your chemotherapy as directed by your oncologist and never use someone else's chemotherapy medications.

Chemotherapy agents can be sorted into two broad categories: (a) Cell-cycle specific agents which affect cells only when they are dividing, and (b) Cell-cycle non-specific agents which affect cells only during their "rest" period (when they are not dividing). The scheduling of chemotherapy is set based on the type of cells, rate at which they divide, and the time at which a given drug is likely to be effective according to the cell cycles. This is why chemotherapy treatment is given in cycles. This means you will go through a period of active treatment followed by a "rest period" (time off from the treatment) before starting another round of treatment. The number of cycles a patient needs is heavily dependent upon the type of cancer, progression of the cancer, and the patient's overall response to the treatments.

Chemotherapy is most effective at killing cells that are rapidly dividing. Unfortunately, chemotherapy agents do not know the difference between your cancerous cells and your normal ones, therefore oftentimes rapidly dividing *healthy* cells will be caught in the crossfire. Fortunately, the normal cells will grow back and be healthy after the treatment is finished; however, in the meantime, side effects will occur as a result of the treatment. The rapidly dividing normal cells commonly affected by chemotherapy are the blood cells, cells in the digestive tract (mouth, stomach, and intestines) and hair follicles. This can result in low blood counts, mouth sores, nausea, diarrhea, and hair loss. Different agents will cause different side effects, depending upon which part of the body is affected. The type of side effects and how strongly they affect the patient depends on many factors:

- The specific type(s) of agent(s) the patient is using.
- Any pre-existing health issues present in the patient.
- Individual metabolism or chemical sensitivities.
- The dosage strength of the chemotherapy agent(s).

- Frequency of chemotherapy treatments.
- Proper use of science-based holistic therapies.

Because of the above-listed factors the side effects experienced will vary from patient to patient, even among those using the same chemotherapy agent. Side effects may include:

- Urine or bowel changes
- Rash or allergic reaction
- Bleeding disorders
- Early menopause
- Nausea/vomiting
- Loss of appetite
- Sun sensitivity
- Organ damage
- Nerve damage
- Skin changes
- Hearing loss
- Hair loss
- Insomnia
- Pain

Each individual chemotherapy agent is associated with certain side effects, so be sure to ask your oncologist for a list of associated side effects for your particular regimen. In the vast majority of cases patients do not experience *all* of the side effects, they only experience some of them. When you do experience any side effects be sure to mention them to your oncologist as well as your holistic practitioners. Most side effects can be reduced through medications as well as holistic methods, and many patients may even use a combination of these. Just be sure that whichever methods you use, let your physicians and practitioners know so that your prescribed treatments and therapies can be adjusted if necessary.

INGREDIENTS

Because there are so many chemotherapy medications available you need to be sure that you are not allergic or intolerant of any of the components that may be in your prescribed agent. For example some chemotherapy medications may contain lactose, others may contain alcohol, and yet others may contain gluten. Others may contain chemical ingredients that you may be allergic to. Be sure your oncologist is fully aware of any allergies or sensitivities you may have before he or she prescribes any chemotherapy agents for you. Likewise, if you choose to use any oral or topical holistic agents be sure the ingredients are compatible with your health. Be sure your practitioner knows if you have any allergies, food sensitivities, or a history of alcoholism.

METHODS OF DELIVERY

Depending upon the agent being use chemotherapy can be administered through the following methods:

- *Oral*: Tablet form or sublingual (under the tongue).
- *Subcutaneous*: Injections under the skin with a hypodermic needle.
- *Intramuscular:* Injections into muscle tissue with a hypodermic needle.
- *Intravenous*: Infusion directly into the bloodstream.
- *Topical*: Applied directly to your skin.
- *Intravesical*: Administered directly into your bladder.
- *Regional*: Applied into the region with the tumor.

Although it would be convenient if all agents could be taken orally, this is not possible: Some agents are rendered ineffective by stomach acids, others are not properly absorbed in the intestines, others are too harsh on the digestive system to be effective, and some just simply work best when administered by the recommended method. Whichever method you are administered, be sure to listen carefully to your oncologist's instructions, get them in writing, and follow them.

HOW TO TAKE YOUR CHEMOTHERAPY AGENTS

Chemotherapy agents which are given through intravenous or regional methods should be administered only by professionals who are licensed to administer such medications. In some cases you may be given a pre-treatment with other medications before your chemotherapy agent in order to prevent certain reactions from happening. As for subcutaneous and intramuscular injections, this depends upon the agent being used; In some cases a licensed professional needs to administer the agent, in other cases a patient can be trained to self-administer the agent. Topical agents are those applied to your skin and are usually prescribed for various types of skin cancer. When using a topical agent be sure that the treatment area is clean and dry before applying. Do not use any other lotions, ointments, creams, essential oils, heat treatments, ultraviolet light therapy or other holistic methods on the treatment site without first discussing it with your doctor as these products may interfere with the efficacy of the agent. Oral medications can usually be taken at home. Some should be taken with food, as the food in your system will slow the transit time that the medication is in you allowing for better absorption of the drug. Some agents on the other hand, should be taken on an *empty stomach*, as food may actually prevent the full absorption of the drug causing you to receive a less than therapeutic dose. In some cases, the presence of food will, instead, result in *too much* absorption of the drug, causing you to develop toxic levels of the drug in your system. Therefore it is extremely important to know if you should be taking your agent with food or an on empty stomach.[44]

---

44 "Empty stomach' means taking the agent at least one hour before eating, or at least 3 hours after eating. When taking on an empty stomach be sure to use only plain water.

DEVELOPING YOUR CHEMOTHERAPY PLAN

Your oncologist will come up with an individualized plan to treat your cancer. Some patients will be treated with only one chemotherapy agent, while other patients may require a combination of agents. In some cases a patient may need a combination of chemotherapy *and* radiation therapy. You need to trust your doctor and stick with his or her plan and this means you need to keep in mind the following:

- No two people will have the same exact care plan for cancer, even if they have the same kind of cancer. This is because treatment plans are based on several factors: The type and progression of the cancer; your age and weight, which other health issues you have, which chemical sensitivities you have, and which other medications you are currently on. This is why your treatment plan will likely vary from someone else's plan even if you both have similar cancers.

- Most chemotherapy drugs can treat more than one kind of cancer, however, none of them can treat *every* kind. Therefore, if your oncologist is not prescribing a certain chemotherapy agent you are interested in then there's a good reason. If you have any questions or concerns then do not be afraid to mention them. Your doctor is your ally in beating this disease, and he or she will gladly answer your questions and address your concerns.

- Some chemotherapy regimens may depend upon whether a patient has had chemotherapy in the past. This is because there are some agents in which only a certain level of lifetime exposure is allowed. If a patient reaches the threshold of this exposure then he or she cannot be allowed to continue with the agent; another agent must be used.

- The genes in your cancer can also make a difference in your treatment regimen. This is because some anti-cancer agents are designed to target specific genes and mutations that are directly involved in the formation of your cancer (a.k.a. "oncogenes"). Therefore your oncologist may order genetic testing of your cancer cells in order to determine your full treatment plan.

When your oncologist creates a chemotherapy plan he or she aims to give you a high enough dose to affect the cancer while trying to keep the side effects to a minimum level. If a combination of agents is necessary then a good doctor will try to avoid giving combinations of multiple agents carrying the same side effects if at all possible. On top of this, the doctor must also be sure that the agents do not interact negatively with each other or with *any other* prescription medications you may be taking. On top of *that*, your doctor also needs to be aware of any vitamins, supplements, or herbs you are taking so that your chemotherapy doesn't negatively react with those either.

Medications, supplements, and herbs are not the only factors considered. Dosage levels are heavily dependent upon a person's body weight and age. Sometimes, depending on the agent, the size of the surface area being treated also makes a difference. Therefore, you can have two patients with the same cancer, but one who is heavier or taller may need a larger dose than the one who is shorter or weighs less. Therefore, if you have any significant weight changes it is important for your oncologist to be aware so that adjustments can be made in your dosages. If, for example, you are an obese man and you lose 75 pounds over the course of your treatment your chemotherapy may become too strong for you and cause you to develop worsening side effects because of it.

As you can see, coming up with an individualized chemotherapy plan for a single patient is a complicated process that is not taken lightly. This is why it is very important to adhere to your doctor's plan.

BRINGING A CHEMOTHERAPY AGENT TO MARKET

Although we still have a long way to go before finding a cure for cancer, medical science has come a long way in finding treatments for destroying tumors, prolonging survival rates and reducing recurrences; this is true of both conventional treatments *and* holistic methods. However, because it can take so long for a single medication to become accepted many cynics believe the pharmaceutical companies are aggressively blocking an actual cancer cure in the interest of money and greed. This is an absurd accusation; in reality, if a company *did* discover an actual *cure* for cancer they would quickly become the wealthiest company in existence as they would hold the sole patent for the cure, causing the entire world to buy the product! The truth is that, just as with any other new medication, in order to provide safe and effective outcomes the researchers are legally obligated to study the proposed medication through a specific sequence of tests and studies before bringing it to the public – this takes many years. Let me give you a brief rundown of what this looks like:

1. **In vitro testing**: This is the first step. It involves taking a cultured sample of human cancer cells and testing the proposed medication or substance directly on these cells without the use of a living organism. This usually takes place in a laboratory using petri dishes, test tubes, or other equipment. Alternatively, researchers may use *ex vivo* testing instead; a process in which they harvest a tissue sample from a living organism and perform the testing directly on the sample. If the in vitro or ex vivo tests show a positive outcome the researchers can progress to *in vivo* testing.

2. **In vivo testing**: This is the point when researchers test the proposed medication or substance on the cancer directly in a living organism. Usually this will involve laboratory mice or rats which are grafted with the human cancer cells and then treated with the proposed medication or substance being researched. Because the law requires medical researchers to perform animal studies as a part of the testing this step cannot be skipped if they hope to bring a medication to market.

This combination of in vitro and in vivo research may take between 3-4 years to complete. If all results show positive outcomes then the scientists can progress to human clinical trials. Before starting human trials the researchers must file an "Investigational New Drug" application with the Food and Drug Administration (FDA). If the FDA does not disapprove of the application within 30 days then the first of the human clinical trials can begin.

3. **Phase 1 Clinical Trial**: Researchers test the new drug in a small group of healthy people (usually up to 80 participants) to evaluate the following: Safe dosage range, method of absorption of the medication in the body, how it is metabolized, how it is distributed through the body, duration of its effect, and how the body excretes it. A Phase 1 trial usually takes 1 year to complete. If results show a positive outcome the research can progress to phase 2.

4. **Phase 2 Clinical Trial**: The new medication is given to a group of patients who have the disease targeted by the medication. Phase 2 studies usually involve a larger number than phase 1 studies and can average up to 300 participants. During this phase the maximum and minimum dosage for effectiveness are evaluated as well as the strength of the medication's effect. A phase 2 trial usually takes about two years to complete. If results show a positive outcome the researchers can progress to phase 3.

5. **Phase 3 Clinical Trial**: This is when the medication is run through the "gold standard" of testing: Randomized, placebo-controlled, double-blind study on a large group of targeted patients; this can involve up to 3,000 participants. During this study the appearance of side effects is noted. A Phase 3 trial usually takes about 3 years to complete.

If results show that Phase 3 has a positive outcome the researchers compile all of the data from these studies and file a "New Drug Application" with the FDA. Because this application will contain all of the research data the document is usually 90 - 100 thousand pages long. The FDA has 60 days to decide whether to review it. Due to the length of the document, if the New Drug Application is approved for review it can take between 2-3 years for the FDA to review it. If the FDA approves of the medication then the researchers can go on to Phase 4.

6. **Phase 4 Clinical Trial**: This is also known as "post-marketing studies." In essence the medication is approved for widespread use and the researchers follow to see if other risks, side-effects, or other unexpected outcomes crop up. Studies are done after the drug or treatment has been marketed to gather information on the drug's effect in various populations and any side effects associated with long-term use. In cases in which the substance shows unexpected dangerous effects it will then be withdrawn from the market.

Following these steps, this means it can take at least *12 years* for a single medication to come to approval – and that is if the drug even makes it through the entire process! On average only 1 in 1,000 investigated medications actually make it to human trials, and of these only a scant few actually make it to market.

Because pharmaceutical companies are required to spend so much time, manpower, and money on a single medication they prefer to spend their resources on medications they *know* they can patent, thus making the enormous efforts worthwhile.

Since natural substances such as herbs, vitamins, and minerals are *not* allowed to be patented most companies avoid putting efforts into them no matter how strong the evidence shows they work. Because these supplements remain untested according to the FDA's standards they cannot be legally sold as medication here in the United States even when legitimate science shows the may be as good – or even better than – the pharmaceuticals that are tested and approved.

Chapter 5
HOLISTIC WAYS TO REDUCE SIDE EFFECTS

Herbs, mushrooms, and supplements listed in this chapter are detailed in chapters 6 and 12 of this book, unless otherwise noted. Other holistic methods listed are described in the appendixes of this book.

ANXIETY & DEPRESSION

Anxiety and depression are common problems for cancer patients, which is really no surprise. The problem is that the anxiety and depression can get in the way of appetite, quality sleep, and quality of life which has the potential to cause other health issues. Yes, there are prescription medications that can be used to alleviate anxiety and depression but since your body is already enduring a chemical assault to destroy the cancer I advise you to first look into non-chemical methods that have been scientifically proven to reduce anxiety and depression such as acupuncture,[45] guided imagery,[46] massage therapy,[47] and music therapy.[48] If you wish to use aromatherapy instead you can try inhaling essential oils such as bergamot, clary sage, English lavender, Roman chamomile, and ylang ylang. Alternatively, if you would prefer herbs and supplements you should ask your practitioner about the use of natural agents such as apigenin, bacopa, bergamot, German chamomile, English lavender, lemon balm, and valerian root. *Precautionary notes*: **(1)** Some practitioners recommend kava kava (*Piper methysticum*) for anxiety, however, this herb is associated with causing severe liver damage, therefore do not use without competent supervision from both your practitioner *and* your oncologist. Do not use if you have a history of liver disease or are on a chemotherapy agent which has the side effect of causing liver damage. **(2)** Some practitioners may also recommend St. John's Wort (*Hypericum perforatum*) for depression; however this herb is well-known for interacting with hundreds of prescription drugs including chemotherapy agents. Be sure you check with your prescribing doctors whether St. John's Wort is compatible with your prescriptions before using.

APPETITE LOSS

Loss of appetite, also known as "anorexia,"[49] may occur due to the side effects of chemotherapy (such as nausea) or from fatigue caused by the disease or the

---

45 *Acupuncture Alleviates Cancer Pain, Fatigue, and Anxiety* (Healthcare Medicine Institute, July 17, 2015)

46 *A Systematic Review of Guided Imagery as an Adjuvant Cancer Therapy.* (Roffe, Schmidt, Ernst, 2005)

47 *The Use of Massage Therapy for Reducing Pain, Anxiety, and Depression in Oncological Palliative Care Patients: A Narrative Review of the Literature.* (Falkensteiner, 2011)

48 *The Effects of Music Therapy on Anxiety and Depression of Cancer Patients.* (Jasemi, 2016)

49 "*Anorexia*" is simple loss of appetite. This is in contrast to "*Anorexia nervosa*", a mental health condition in which a person purposely starves him or herself in the belief that he or she is overweight.

treatments themselves. Any loss of appetite during cancer treatment needs to be addressed quickly because without proper nutrition and sufficient fluid intake your body will not have the resources it needs in order to fight the cancer. If you are having a difficult time mustering up your appetite you may want to try eating small, nutritious meals several times throughout the day instead of three regular meals; just be sure you are taking in your required calorie count for the day as established by your doctor or dietitian. Suggestions for small meals include (but are not limited to):

- Whole grain crackers or toast with cheese or peanut butter
- Sardines or tuna with whole grain crackers or toast
- English muffin with peanut butter or egg
- Apples or celery with peanut butter or cheese
- Tortilla chips with refried beans and salsa
- Yogurt topped with granola and berries
- Whole grain chips with guacamole
- Pretzels with hummus
- Home made trail mix
- Finger sandwiches

If you cannot eat a small meal try to snack healthy all day while aiming for your calorie goal. Suggested snacks may include hard boiled eggs, cheese pieces, yogurt cups, sunflower or pumpkin seeds, roasted soy beans or chick peas, sliced meats, nuts, kale chips, fresh fruit and vegetable pieces, dehydrated fruits and vegetables, whole grain breads, a handful of whole grain cold cereal, and whole grain crackers. Stay away from empty calories such as cookies, candy, sodas, etc. because you need nutrient-dense foods to keep your stamina while you fight this disease. If you must have a sweet snack keep in mind that certain dehydrated fruits such as pineapple, raisins, apples, and strawberries can tame a sugar craving while delivering better nutrition than candy. Alternatively you can make healthy smoothies in the blender: Start with a protein base such as yogurt, milk, silken tofu, high protein vegan milks, etc. Add your frozen fruits and/or chopped vegetables and enough water or ice to liquefy. Another option is to make a healthy, home made soup and process it in the blender to make it a drinkable soup. If you choose this option be aware that meat should be diced small in order to blend well.

You must also be sure you are getting sufficient fluids throughout the day. Not only does this help prevent nausea but it also prevents illness caused by dehydration *and* helps your body flush out the chemotherapy agents properly so they do not build up toxic levels in your system (which increases the side effects). Fluids include almost anything that is liquid at room temperature such as water, juice, frozen juice bars, decaffeinated coffee or tea, gelatin, ice chips, milk, nutritional shakes, and breakfast drinks. Avoid beverages with alcohol or caffeine as these substances tend to promote dehydration by drawing water out of your system.

If, in spite of the above information, you are still not reaching your daily calorie goals I advise you to speak with a competent herbalist regarding the use of appetite stimulators such as bergamot, bitter greens, cannabis sativa, scaly wood mushroom, and papaya. If cannabis sativa is not legal in your area ask your doctor about using legal prescription medications which contain cannabinoids that may increase your appetite. Alternatively, you may choose to speak with a licensed acupuncturist as studies have proven acupuncture to be a useful in increasing appetite in cancer patients.[50]

CHEMO BRAIN

One well-known complication of chemotherapy is a condition known as "Chemo brain" a.k.a chemotherapy-related cognitive impairment, or cognitive dysfunction. Chemo brain is a side effect of chemotherapy which may cause memory lapses, trouble with multi-tasking, forgetfulness, decreased ability to concentrate, slower thinking response, and trouble remembering words, names, dates, etc. It is often a side effect caused by the toxic effects of chemotherapy. For most people this effect can come on quickly but is only temporary (usually going away soon after chemotherapy treatments are completed). Fortunately, this side effect does not happen to everyone. Although, at this time, science doesn't *fully* understand the process, studies have revealed certain situations which tend to increase the chances of developing chemo brain, such as:

- The presence of certain other health issues aside from the cancer
- Hormone treatments or hormonal changes
- Infections or other underlying disease
- Nutritional deficiencies
- Certain medications
- Surgical anesthesia
- Fatigue, insomnia
- Low blood counts
- Stress or anxiety
- Depression
- Age

There are several ways you can cope with chemo brain as you undergo your treatments. Many patients make use of a day-planner, whether it is a little book to keep in your pocket or a calendar on your device. You can also help yourself by exercising your brain: Do some word puzzles, learn some phrases in a new language, take an art class – anything to keep your thinking "muscles" going. If you are not too fatigued from your treatments you should also try light exercise; something easy to keep you moving such as walking, biking, marching in place, stretching, or anything that you are physically able to do. Not only does exercise increase mental alertness but can also improve the quality of your sleep – which is also known to increase

---

50 Cancer-associated Anorexia and Cachexia in Adults with GI Tract Cancer: Novel Intervention with Acupuncture. (Yoon, 2014) [Presented at: Oncology Nursing Society 39th Congress, May 1-5, 2014, Anaheim, CA]

mental alertness. If you are home bound and cannot get out to exercise or take classes then I advise you to speak to your practitioners about herbs such as guarana and bacopa,[51] or the essential oil of rosemary.[52] Although antioxidants are also well-known for helping to reduce chemo-brain it is important to remember that many chemotherapy agents are weakened by the use of antioxidants. Therefore, I strongly suggest that you consult with your oncologist *first* before using antioxidant supplements. Antioxidants commonly used for reducing chemo-brain include n-Acetyl cysteine, Coenzyme Q-10, and lecithin.

CHEMOTHERAPY RESISTANCE

One common obstacle during chemotherapy treatment is situations in which the cancer develops a resistance to the chemotherapy agent, a.k.a. "tachyphylaxis," resulting in the slow-down of any progress. This resistance happens when the cancer cells begin to make a substance known as p-glycoprotein which helps them prevent absorption of the chemotherapy agents into their membranes. When this happens your choices are to **(1)** get the cancer re-sensitized to the agent or **(2)**, switch to a different agent or combination of agents to fight the disease. Some chemotherapy agents are more likely to find resistance than others, such as paclitaxel, doxorubicin, vincristine, and others. Ask your oncologist if any of the agents you are taking are known for developing resistance. If you do find that your cancer has become resistant your oncologist may offer you some prescription medications to help counteract this situation. Alternatively you may consult with an experienced herbal practitioner regarding anti-resistance herbs and supplements such as: Asian ginseng, berberine, beta-elemine, emodin, evodiamine, licorice root, omega 3 fatty acids, piperine, resveratrol, and quercetin (all of which are detailed in chapter 6 of this book). Be sure you discuss this alternative supplementation with your oncologist before making the changes.

CONSTIPATION

Constipation occurs when the bowels are too sluggish to move waste through, or when the waste itself is too compacted and too hard to move through properly.

Sluggish bowels are primarily caused by prescription painkillers, sedentary lifestyles, and the use of iron supplements. One of the most natural ways to relieve constipation caused by sluggish bowels is by daily performing half an hour of gentle exercise, such as walking, stretching, bicycling, or water exercises. The action of regular exercise stimulates your muscles to help pass stool through the bowel. Another natural way to relieve sluggish bowels is to consume insoluble fiber foods as these provide the roughage which helps push material through the bowel. Insoluble

---

51 Although some practitioners may also recommend ginkgo biloba for chemo-brain, there are no current studies supporting this herb for this particular condition. In fact, one study observed that ginkgo did not prevent chemo-brain in test subjects: *The use of Ginkgo biloba for the prevention of chemotherapy-related cognitive dysfunction in women receiving adjuvant treatment for breast cancer, N00C9.* (Barton, 2013)

52 *Plasma 1,8-Cineole Correlates with Cognitive Performance Following Exposure to Rosemary Essential Oil Aroma* (Moss and Oliver, 2003)

fiber foods include bran cereals, raw or dried fruits and vegetables, (with skins on when possible), prunes, and whole grains.[53] Avoid eating large amounts of cheese, bananas, and refined grains as these tend to move slowly through the bowel. Eat at least two servings of high fiber foods per meal if you do not have bowel disease. If you do have bowel disease (whether cancer-related or not) you must discuss any use of fiber with your treating physician first.

To combat constipation caused by hard compacted stool you should increase your fluid intake in order to soften the stool thus allowing it to pass through naturally. You may also try increasing your intake of foods with soluble fiber, which is an indigestible carbohydrate that absorbs water. The absorption of this water into your stool will help soften it and allow it to pass through. Common foods containing soluble fiber include fruits and vegetables, oatmeal, and legumes (beans, peas, lentils). Make sure you drink plenty of water with the foods in order for the fiber to work properly. Alternatively, you may also want to speak to your doctor about the use of exercise, magnesium supplements, or bromelain supplements to help the soluble fiber do its job.

DIARRHEA

Diarrhea happens when your bowel is unable to absorb water from the digested material received from the small intestine. This inability to absorb the fluid may be caused by injury to the bowel lining (either through disease or chemotherapy agents) or by an overstimulated bowel that passes the digested matter through too quickly to allow for proper fluid absorption.

Not only can diarrhea be inconvenient and embarrassing, but it can also be painful and physically irritating. On top of this, if the diarrhea is severe enough it can cause severe health problems due to the dehydration caused by the lack of fluid resorption into the body. Therefore, if you begin to experience bouts of diarrhea during your treatment you must let your doctor and other practitioners know so the problem can be quickly addressed.

Oftentimes the avoidance of certain foods may help reduce bouts of diarrhea. This may include eliminating menu items such as high fatty foods, dairy products, spicy foods, and anything containing alcohol or caffeine. It is also wise to avoid tobacco products and alcohol sugars.[54]

Balancing the flora in your bowel may also help (flora is the beneficial micro-organisms necessary for a healthy bowel). This can be achieved by taking probiotic supplements or eating fermented foods with active cultures. Fermented foods include menu items such as kefir, kimchi, kombucha, kvass, miso, natto, raw cheese, rejuvelac, sauerkraut, seed cheese, tempeh, and yogurt. Take note of three important facts: **(1)** Using fermented foods and probiotics daily may take up to two weeks to

---

53 Whole grains are unrefined which means they contain all parts of the entire kernel. These include: Amaranth, buckwheat, bulgur, corn, cracked wheat, quinoa, brown rice, popcorn, sorghum, spelt, wheat berries, whole wheat wild rice, and any grain or flour labeled as "whole." If you follow a gluten free diet then you should avoid the following: Barley, bulgur, durum, einkorn, emmer, farro, freekeh/frika, kamut, rye, semolina, spelt, triticale, wheat, and wheat berries.

54 "Alcohol sugars" are any sweeteners with the suffix "-itol" such as sorbitol, mannitol, xylitol, etc.

achieve full effect. **(2)** Fermented foods which are heated or cooked, such as sourdough bread, etc., will kill the probiotic effect rendering it useless. **(3)** "Pickles" are often referred to as fermented, however there is a catch: Any pickle listing "vinegar" in the ingredients are *not* fermented; you will need to seek out pickles which are made without vinegar. These are usually found in natural food stores and specialty shops.

Another method to alleviate diarrhea is by using bulking agents. These are over-the-counter products made with methylcellulose fiber which absorb water in the bowel, thereby solidifying the stool and reducing bouts of diarrhea. Be sure you drink a full glass of water with these agents in order for them to work effectively. Do not use bulking agents without discussing it with your physician first, especially if you have any kind of bowel disease.

You should also keep track of your intake of electrolytes. Electrolytes are water-soluble nutrients such as potassium, calcium, magnesium, and sodium that are essential for normal function of the heart and your muscles. The loss of fluid brought on by diarrhea can result in dangerously low electrolyte levels which can cause death. Be aware, though, that too many electrolytes in your system may also cause adverse health issues. Therefore I strongly advise you speak with your physician regarding your electrolyte intake requirements.

FAMILY PLANNING

For Women: Because chemotherapy is such a strong treatment you should be sure to let your oncologist know immediately if you are already pregnant. Chemotherapy is extremely damaging to an unborn child and will cause the child's death. Pregnant patients need a specialized plan in order to protect the unborn child as much as possible. If you are not pregnant, DO NOT GET PREGNANT UNTIL YOUR DOCTOR SAYS IT IS SAFE. Depending upon the treatment used this may require a period of waiting for several months *after* treatment before planning a child, just to be safe. If you remain sexually active during your treatment be sure to use *two* forms of birth control each time to reduce the chances of an unplanned pregnancy. If you are not pregnant but are breastfeeding you need to be aware that your chemotherapy agents may come through your breast milk. This can severely hurt or kill your baby, therefore I strongly advise against any breastfeeding until your doctor says it is safe. Although breastfeeding is touted as the best thing for your baby, know that chemotherapy agents are the *worst* thing for your little one. This is one of those times you need to switch to baby formula or hire a trusted wet nurse. Depending upon the treatment used it may be a period of several weeks *after* finishing treatment before it is safe to breastfeed again. Discuss this with your oncologist. In order to maintain milk production during your chemotherapy treatments be sure to use a breast pump several times a day and pour the milk down the drain. When your doctor tells you it is safe to breastfeed again immediately throw away the pump, as it may be contaminated with chemotherapy residue, and use a new one for your baby.

For Men: Men should be informed that many chemotherapy agents can seriously affect sperm production resulting in severely defective sperm; therefore you should not father children until your oncologist says it is safe. Other chemotherapy agents can absorb into the semen and pose a toxic risk to your partner, therefore men should refrain from direct sexual contact with their partners throughout the duration of those treatments. Be sure to speak to your oncologist regarding safety precautions in handling the agents and during sexual contact.

For Both: It also important to be aware that there are some particular chemotherapy agents which can cause permanent infertility in either men or women, depending upon the agent. If you and your mate desire to have children after your treatments are finished be sure you speak to your oncologist about the risks of infertility. Females can discuss the option of storing their eggs or storing ovarian tissue and males can discuss the option of storing their sperm for later family planning. Couples may also discuss the option of freezing their embryos for later implantation, hiring a surrogate mother, or adoption.

FATIGUE

Fatigue during cancer treatment can come from the different treatments, the cancer itself, or the exhaustion from the entire ordeal. Oftentimes cancer-related fatigue continues for a while even after treatments are finished, this is not abnormal since your body needs some serious recovery time after having fought off cancer. To help reduce bouts of fatigue it is best to simply not push yourself any more than is necessary. Make sure you give yourself regular rest intervals and do not feel obligated to commit to activities or events that are not essential. You should also make sure you drink plenty of fluids and eat a healthy diet; avoid foods which are over-processed, fried, fatty, or heavy with artificial ingredients.

If this is not enough to combat fatigue you may want to try other methods such as acupuncture,[55] or aromatherapeutic agents such as oils of black pepper, grapefruit, jasmine, and lemon. If you prefer to use herbs and supplements you should consult with your practitioner regarding the use of American ginseng, Asian ginseng, bu zhong yi qi, cordyceps, ganoderma, and guarana.

HAIR LOSS

There are not a lot of remedies for chemotherapy induced hair loss, let me explain why: Cancer cells replicate much faster than healthy cells; this is why chemotherapy agents target fast replicating cells. The problem is that, even though *most* of your healthy body cells replicate slower, not all of them are so slow: hair follicles are among the faster ones. Ergo, when certain chemotherapy agents are killing fast replicating cells the hair follicles sometimes get caught in the crossfire. The good news is that not all chemotherapy treatments result in hair loss, however, if you are put on a regimen with an agent which causes hair loss do not let this discourage you as there are at least a couple of methods in which patients have reported to be successful, such as cold cap therapy and certain herbs and supplements.

---

55 *Acupuncture Alleviates Cancer Pain, Fatigue, and Anxiety* (Healthcare Medicine Institute, July 17, 2015)

Cold Cap Therapy: This is a method of treatment which was approved by the FDA in 2015 for reducing hair loss caused by certain chemotherapy treatments. The cold cap system works by cooling the patient's scalp to near-freezing temperatures. This tends to slow the blood flow into the scalp which in turn slows the flow of intravenous chemotherapy medications to the scalp, thus reducing the amount of the agents reaching the hair follicles. The reduction in medication reaching the follicles translates into a reduction in hair loss. When using a cold cap therapy you will need to keep your scalp cooled before, during, and after your dose of chemotherapy. You should be aware that you may still sustain some hair loss, and the hair you do retain may become more dry or brittle. During this time do not use hair dyes, perms, or other harsh chemicals. When you finish your chemotherapy series your hair should grow back normally. Be aware that not all patients are suitable for this treatment, especially those who have health issues with scalp.

Herbs and Supplements: Some patients have reported success with using Active Hexose Correlated Compound (AHCC), a commercial product made with medicinal mushroom extracts. Studies have shown that this compound can reduce hair loss caused by treatment with the chemotherapy agent cytosine arabinoside.[56] Others have had success with using selenium supplements, a natural mineral found in several foods. Use caution with selenium though as this mineral can become very toxic if overused; do not consume more than 400mcg (micrograms) total per day. Keep in mind that certain foods, especially Brazil nuts, are very high in the mineral. I strongly advise that you take it only with professional supervision.

If you find that you are not suitable for cold cap treatment or the suggested herbs and supplements you may want to consider the following:

- Hair does not always fall out evenly, therefore you may want to cut your hair shorter in order to hide balding spots more effectively.
- You may want to cut your hair and have a wig made from it. Being it is your own natural hair it will be an exact color match for you and it will look, feel, and "act" more like regular hair than a wig. You will need at least 6 inches of hair length to make a wig.
- Some insurance companies will pay for a wig if it is prescribed by a doctor (prescribed as a "cranial prosthesis"). It is better to get your wig while you still have some hair so the stylist can see your hair and get the best match for you if you do not use your own hair.
- If you are in need of a wig and your insurance will not cover it you can contact your local chapters of the American Cancer Society, CancerCare, or Susan G. Komen for the Cure and inquire about their cancer wig programs. Oftentimes you may be able to receive a wig at no charge.

Also, be aware that hair loss caused by chemotherapy treatments is usually reversible, meaning your hair will grow back once the treatments are finished. One exception is with the chemotherapy drug docetaxel, a.k.a. Taxotere; this agent is known for causing permanent hair loss.

---

56 *The Effect of Active Hexose Correlated Compound in Modulating Cytosine Arabinoside-induced Hair Loss, and 6-mercaptopurine -and-methotrexate-induced Liver Injury in Rodents.* (Sun, 2009)

HAND FOOT SYNDROME

Hand Foot Syndrome, also known to as Palmar-Plantar Erythrodysesthesia, is one of the side effects experienced by a small percentage of chemotherapy patients. Some chemotherapy agents run a higher risk of this side effect than others; consult with your oncologist. Symptoms develop in the hands and feet, oftentimes with any combination of pain, tingling, burning, numbness, reddening, swelling, blisters, sores, and peeling of the skin. This condition results when a chemotherapy agent becomes congested in the hands in feet causing them to leak from the tiny blood vessels into the flesh of the outer extremities. Prevention is key when trying to reduce the development of hand-foot syndrome. Doctors often give the following good advice to help reduce the risk of developing this side effect:

- Reduce exposure to heat or friction on your hands and feet during your treatments and for seven days afterward.
- Elevate your arms and legs after each treatment to help prevent congestion of the chemotherapy agent in the extremities.
- Do not allow hands or feet to remain in hot water (washing dishes, long showers, etc.). When showering, use lukewarm instead of hot water. No tub baths.
- When cleaning do not use rubber or plastic gloves; do not use harsh chemicals.
- Avoid any unnecessary pressure on hands or feet (excessive standing, weight lifting, jogging, etc.)
- Avoid using sharp implements to reduce the risk of cuts.
- Avoid using hand tools whenever possible.
- Do not allow foot or hand massages until your doctor says it is okay.
- Avoid extreme hot or cold temperatures on your hands and feet.
- Use ice packs wrapped in a layer of cloth on your hands and feet in twenty minute intervals during treatment to reduce the amount of chemotherapy agent being circulated into those extremities (a similar principle used in cold cap therapy, see the subheading "Hair Loss" in this chapter).

If you have already developed hand and foot syndrome there are still ways you can lessen the discomfort such as wrapping ice cold packs in a cloth and apply to the affected sites for twenty minute intervals, and pat yourself dry after a shower instead of rubbing. Many patients also find some relief by applying aloe vera gel, henna paste, or marshmallow root infusion to the affected areas. For your laundry use unscented, dye free products and always put your loads through an extra rinse cycle to remove any detergent residues. When experiencing symptoms keep in mind that broken or peeling skin may run the risk of infections; monitor for any formation of pus, excessive swelling or hot, red, painful skin. Try to look for hygiene products made of all-natural ingredients from companies such as Tom's of Maine, Weleda, Burt's Bees, and J.R. Watkins, among others. Instead of using harsh chemicals during your house cleaning use all-natural products, or scrub with baking soda. Do not use vinegar as it is painful on raw, broken skin.

HEARING LOSS[57]

Hearing loss caused by chemotherapy may be temporary or permanent. Agents associated with causing hearing loss include bleomycin, bromocriptine, carboplatin, cisplatin, cyclophosphamide, mechlorethamine, methotrexate, vinblastine, and vincristine. Each agent has its own level of risk so you will need to discuss this with your oncologist. Signs of hearing loss include: Ringing in the ears, buzzing sounds, pulsing sounds, ear pain, nausea, and dizziness. Hearing loss sometimes continues even after treatment has been finished, and usually it is the ability to hear high-frequency sound that is affected. A patient's risk of developing hearing loss is often (but not always) tied to one's individual genetics. Studies have shown that mutations in the WFS1 gene[58] and the ACYP2[59] and patients with Cockayne syndrome[60] are heavily associated with a higher risk of cisplatin-induced hearing loss.

Although there are some are some prescription medications which may help reduce the risk of hearing loss associated with chemotherapy some patients have had good results using supplements such as alpha-lipoic acid, melatonin and low doses of resveratrol to help reduce this side effect. For the sake of protecting your sense of hearing I strongly advise that you do not self-treat; use these supplements only under the supervision of your oncologist *and* your holistic practitioner.

HEART BURN

Heartburn occurs when the valve between the esophagus and your stomach does not close properly, thus allowing some of the acidic stomach contents to back up into the esophagus; this can be caused by tumor interference, obesity, or weakness caused by cancer treatments. One of the best ways to reduce bouts of heartburn is by modifying your diet: Remove caffeinated products, alcoholic beverages, high fatty foods, chocolate, and highly acidic foods from your meals as these all promote more acid production. It is also beneficial to follow a vegan diet as the plant proteins are much easier to digest than the tougher animal-based proteins. Just be sure you consult with a nutritionist or registered dietitian[61] first to ensure you are meeting your daily protein requirements. If you tend to experience heartburn when lying down you should try laying on your left side or use pillows or a bed wedge to prop your upper body up higher than your lower body to prevent stomach acids from backing up into your esophagus.

Herbs and supplements: Some of the most effective items to reduce heartburn include baking soda, calcium,[62] carob, or marshmallow root infusion. Although

---

57 Hearing loss caused by chemotherapy agents is often referred to as "ototoxicity."

58 *Variants in WFS1 and other Mendelian deafness genes are associated with cisplatin-associated ototoxicity* (Wheeler, 2016)

59 *Replication of a genetic variant in ACYP2 associated with cisplatin-induced hearing loss in patients with osteosarcoma.* (Vos, 2016)

60 *Mutations in Cockayne Syndrome-associated Genes (Csa and Csb) Predispose to Cisplatin-induced Hearing Loss in Mice.* (Rainey, 2016)

61 Both nutritionists and registered dietitians are educated in diet, food and nutrition, *however* dietitians are required to have a college education whereas nutritionists are not.

62 Do not use calcium products which contain acids (such as calcium fortified orange juice) or fats (such as milk or cheeses) as the acids and fats will worsen your heartburn. Instead use a chewable

peppermint and ginger can be used to counteract nausea do not use them for heartburn because they may make it worse.

INSOMNIA

Insomnia is a common problem for cancer patients. It can be caused by anxiety, the cancer treatments, or by other medications not related to the cancer. First, check with your prescribing physicians to see if any of your prescription medications contain caffeine or other substances that may interfere with sleep. If they do you should discuss either changing medications or switching the time of day you take your medications. You should also be aware of any herbs or supplements that you may be taking as they may also contribute to insomnia. Herbs such as guarana, yerba mate, and cola nut contain caffeine, and other herbs such as ginger, rosemary, and mint tend to have other stimulating properties. Note also that beverages such as cocoa, tea, coffee and some sodas also contain caffeine. If medications, supplements, and beverages are not the problem there are still things you can do to get better sleep. For example:

Darkness: When it is time for sleep make sure your bedroom is as dark as possible. Darkness induces your body to make melatonin, a hormone which helps regulate your sleep cycle. Buy room-darkening shades and curtains if you need to, especially if you have street lights or business lights shining into your window, or if you are a night worker that needs to sleep during the daytime. Be aware that low light such as night lights or digital clock lights may also disrupt sleep; therefore unplug the night light and turn your clock away from you.

Diet: Do not eat at least three hours before sleep, as digestion tends to take a lot of energy resulting in an increased metabolism which prevents your body from slowing down to rest. Also, you should avoid anything with caffeine or energy drinks for at least *six* hours before sleep to make sure any caffeine or other energizing substance is out of your system.

Exercise: Although you should not exercise within 3 hours before bedtime (because it increases your metabolism, making it harder to sleep) you should get some regular exercise every day as your energy level allows. Studies have shown that getting at least 25 minutes of exercise per day promotes a more healthful, restful sleep. Therefore, be sure you get your exercise, just make sure you do it early in the day.

Bedtime Routine: If you do not already have a bedtime routine, make one now. Start an hour before bedtime by changing into your pajamas and brushing your teeth. Then dim the lights to prime your mind and body for rest. Turn off the television and do something relaxing for the remainder of the hour: Listen to soothing music, do some light reading, engage in a guided imagery session, spend time in prayer, etc.

Holistic methods: Acupuncture has been shown to be as good, if not better, than sleeping pills with the bonus of having none of the side effects that the pills

---

calcium supplement or calcium based antacid tablet. Take note that calcium may interfere with the absorption of some prescriptions, speak to your doctor first.

have.[63] For those who prefer aromatherapy, certain essential oils such as English lavender, Roman chamomile, and sweet marjoram are well-known for promoting sleep. If, instead, you prefer to use herbal teas then speak with your herbalist about using plants with proven sedative effects such as valerian root, lemon balm, and German chamomile.

MOUTH SORES

Some chemotherapy agents may cause sores to form on the inner lips, cheeks, tongue, gums, and throat; oftentimes this causes patients to put off oral hygiene due to the discomfort. Patients who are dealing with mouth sores should start with switching to a soft-bristled toothbrush to lessen the irritation on the sores. Instead of using commercial toothpastes you should try plain baking soda sprinkled onto the wet toothbrush no more than three times per week. For patients who do not want to use baking soda they can still brush with a soft toothbrush and plain water, just be sure to follow it with a mild, antiseptic mouth rinse afterward. Alternatively, you may wrap your finger in a washcloth, wet the cloth and gently scrub your teeth with it. Patients who wear braces, dentures, retainers, or partial plates may have difficulty because the sores make their oral appliances uncomfortable to wear or the appliances may make the sores worse. I advise speaking with your dentist or orthodontist to discuss your options.

If this is not enough to give you relief you may want to speak to your practitioner about using herbal-based mouth rinses made from calendula, German chamomile, or marshmallow root.

Precautionary notes: Some practitioners also recommend arnica, however arnica can be toxic when swallowed, therefore I do not promote its use as a mouth rinse. Some may also recommend slippery elm (bark), however, harvesting the bark from the trees effectively kills the trees and as a result the tree is now endangered, therefore I also do not recommend using slippery elm.

NAUSEA / VOMITING

Nausea and vomiting is a common issue for patients during chemotherapy treatments. If you find this to be a problem you might want to start with modifying your diet: Consume easy-to-digest foods such as applesauce, white rice, white toast, vegetable proteins, saltine crackers, water, and plain black tea. If this is not enough to tame the nausea you may opt for using aromatherapeutics such as the essential oils of peppermint, spearmint, or ginger as inhalant therapy. Alternatively you may wish to consult with a licensed acupuncturist, as this method has been shown to reduce nausea in cancer patients by a whopping 49%.[64] If you prefer to use herbs and supplements you should speak to your practitioner about using herbs proven to reduce nausea such as cannabis sativa,[65] cloves, ginger, hot peppers, peppermint, scaly wood mushrooms, or spearmint.

---

63 *Acupuncture For the Treatment of Insomnia* (Zhao, 2013)

64 *Acupuncture Alleviates Cancer Pain, Fatigue, and Anxiety* (Healthcare Medicine Institute, July 17, 2015)

65 This herb is not legal in all areas of the country. If you cannot legally use it in your location speak to your doctor about a prescription for cannabis based medications that are legal to use.

NERVE DAMAGE

Nerve damage, also known as neuropathy, is commonly associated with chemotherapy agents such as bortezomib, docetaxel, epothilones, paclitaxel, platinum agents, thalidomide, and vincristine. Symptoms of neuropathy may include numbness, tingling, sensations of heat or cold, or pain, especially in the hands and feet. This condition may not always be reversible therefore a strongly advise you to speak with your oncologist regarding the steps you can take to reduce the risk. If you are already experiencing any of these symptoms be sure to tell your oncologist as he or she may be able to make adjustments in your treatment to reduce the potential for further damage.

Herbs and supplements known to help reduce the severity of neuropathy include milk thistle, German chamomile extract, ginkgo biloba, Vitamins B6 and B12 combined, L-carnitine, sweet bee venom, and alpha-lipoic acid. Chinese herbal formulas such as Buyang Huanhu,[66] and Chaihu Long Gumuli Wan,[67] (which are not described in chapter 6 of this book) have also been shown to be clinically relevant.

Precautionary note: Many herbs used to counteract neuropathy contains antioxidants. Because some cancer therapies depend on oxidation to destroy cancer be sure you speak with your oncologist before using any of the listed items.

ORGAN DAMAGE

Some chemotherapy agents are known for increased risk of damage to vital organs such as the heart, liver, kidneys, and lungs. Oftentimes chemotherapy-induced organ damage can be reduced or prevented by the use of antioxidants, however, some chemotherapy agents are weakened by the excessive use of antioxidants. Therefore I strongly advise you to discuss this with your oncologist before starting on an antioxidant regimen.

Heart damage, also known as cardiomyopathy, is commonly associated with anthracyclines, cyclophosphamide, mitoxantrone, paclitaxel, and trastuzumab. Take note that the higher the dose of treatments, the higher the risk of developing heart damage – and sometimes these effects may take several months to show. It is also worth noting that patients with a BRCA gene mutation (related to certain kinds of breast cancer) tend to experience a higher risk of developing heart damage with chemotherapy. One study noted that combining radiation treatments with doxorubicin increases the risk of cardiomyopathy[68] while another study observed that combining trastuzumab with paclitaxel after doxorubicin and cyclophosphamide also carried a high risk of developing heart damage.[69] Herbs known to help reduce heart damage

---

66 *Buyang Huanhu Decoction in Prevention of Peripheral Neuropathy After Chemotherapy: A Clinical Observation.* (Sun, 2008)

67 *Combined Application of Traditional Chinese Medicine Prevention of Taxol Chemotherapy-induced Peripheral Neuropathy: A Clinical Observation.* (Pan, 2012)

68 *Pathophysiological effects of radiation on atherosclerosis development and progression, and the incidence of cardiovascular complications* (Basavaraju, 2002)

69 *Assessment of Cardiac Dysfunction in a Randomized Trial Comparing Doxorubicin and Cyclophosphamide Followed by Paclitaxel, With or Without Trastuzumab, as Adjuvant Therapy in Node-Positive Human Epidermal Growth Factor Receptor 2 – Overexpressing Breast Cancer: NSABP B-31 (* Tan-Chiu, 2005)

include milk thistle, baikal skullcap, grape seed extract, and Acetyl L-carnitine.

Liver damage, a.k.a. hepatotoxicity, is associated with asparaginase, nitrosureas, antimetabolites, vinca alkaloids, cisplatin and cyclophosphamide. Liver damage is usually mild and reversible, though it may contribute to cirrhosis of the liver later in life. Because many other prescription medications are processed through the liver you may need to speak to your prescribing physician's about changing your medications, including over-the- counter products, if you are required to use a chemotherapy agent known to risk liver damage. The lesser the amount of chemicals being processed through your liver, the lesser the risk of damage sustained. Herbs and supplements that may help protect your liver include: Active Hexose Correlated Compound, Milk thistle, acetyl L-carnitine, milk thistle, dandelion, tamalaki, haoqin qingdan, thymoquinone, and grape seed extract.

Kidney damage, also known as nephrotoxicity, is commonly associated with agents such as cisplatin, oxaliplatin, carboplatin,[70] nitrosureas, mitomycin, and methotrexate. When using an agent which carries a risk to your kidneys make sure you are drinking enough fluids each day during treatment to help flush the agent through your system efficiently. Speak to your doctor about lowering your salt intake as salt tends to hold fluids inside your body instead of letting them be released. Diabetic patients should be especially vigilant concerning their kidneys as diabetes in itself can be very damaging to the kidneys. Milk thistle extract is known to protect the kidneys from chemo-based damage and should be given *just before* the chemotherapy agent is administered. Other herbs known to reduce kidney damage include ginger, resveratrol, magnesium, grape seed extract and black cumin combined with German chamomile.

Lung damage, a.k.a. pulmonary toxicity, or scarring of the lungs, is usually associated with arsenic trioxide, bleomycin, and idarubicin. If you are using an agent with a risk to the lungs you absolutely must quit smoking all substances (tobacco, clove cigarettes, marijuana, etc.) and stay out of polluted and dusty areas as much as you reasonably can, including smoke filled rooms. You may want to speak to your physician about using a device called an incentive spirometer, which is a hand-held tool which exercises your lungs and promotes deep breathing.

PAIN

Whether pain is caused by the cancer itself or by chemotherapy effects pain is sometimes a real concern for some patients. Although there are prescription pain killers these can cause other problems such as liver or kidney stress and constipation, not to mention that some patients are sensitive or even allergic to such medications. Fortunately, several forms of holistic methods have been proven to significantly reduce pain in cancer patients. For example, acupuncture has been shown to reduce cancer pain by 51%,[71] massage therapy has been observed to reduce pain for up to 18

---

70 Research has shown that kidney damage can happen within one hour of receiving platinum-based agents.

71 *Acupuncture Alleviates Cancer Pain, Fatigue, and Anxiety* (Healthcare Medicine Institute, July 17, 2015)

hours,[72] music therapy has also been shown to significantly reduce cancer-related pain,[73] and guided imagery has also been successful in reducing pain in cancer patients. If you prefer to use plant-based therapies you should speak to your practitioner about the use of herbs and supplements such as bacopa, boswellia, bromelain, cannabis sativa,[74] devil's claw, ginger, papaya/papain, and white willow bark. Remember to speak with your oncologist before using herbal methods to ensure they do not clash with your chemotherapy agents.

RED BLOOD CELLS

Oftentimes chemotherapy suppresses the bone marrow's ability to manufacture red and white blood cells. Like hair follicles, bone cells are also fast replicators (this is necessary for making blood cells). Since chemotherapy agents target fast replicating cells your bone and blood cells sometimes get caught up in the crossfire causing suppression of your blood cells. Your oncologist may want to prescribe iron supplements to help you build up your red blood cells, however these supplements are notorious for causing constipation and iron can become toxic if overused. It is also important to take note that using iron supplements during therapy with anthracyclines may increase the risk of chemotherapy-induced heart damage. If you prefer to avoid the iron supplements you may wish to speak with both your oncologist and a competent herbalist about using iron-rich herbal methods such as scaly wood mushroom or yellow dock root to boost your iron needs.

You may, instead, decide that you'd rather boost your iron levels through diet alone. If you choose to use an iron-rich diet for your supplementation be sure you consult with a registered dietitian or a competent nutritionist to ensure you are keeping to a balanced diet.

SECOND CANCERS

Do not confuse "second cancer" with "*secondary cancer.*" A *secondary cancer* is an original cancer which has metastasized elsewhere in your body. In contrast, a "second cancer" is another cancer that is different from the original cancer. Some chemotherapy agents may increase the risk of developing a second cancer later in life. For example, a woman given alkylating agents during her breast cancer treatment is at a higher risk of developing leukemia later in her life. This is not a common side effect but it is important to understand that it does happen from time to time. Be sure you discuss with your oncologist whether your chemotherapy regimen carries this risk as it is important for you to know to watch out for symptoms later in life if you do happen to be one of the few who develop a second cancer.

Because the risk of developing a second cancer is rather small, and is extremely variable from person to person, any holistic methods would need to be used

---

72 *The Use of Massage Therapy for Reducing Pain, Anxiety, and Depression in Oncological Palliative Care Patients: A Narrative Review of the Literature.* (Falkensteiner, 2011)

73 *Effect of Music Therapy on Pain and Anxiety Levels of Cancer Patients: A Pilot Study.* (Krishnaswamy, 2016)

74 This herb is not legal in all areas of the country. If you cannot legally use it in your location speak to your doctor about a prescription for cannabis based medications that are legal to use.

on a case by case basis. However, if you wish to reduce your risk of developing a second cancer to begin with here is some general advice: Eliminate all tobacco and alcohol products from your life. Work yourself into a vegan diet and try to eat as much organic and natural food as you can afford on your budget. The less processed the food, the better – also stay away from food additives and preservatives. Cut out high fatty foods, keep your sugar consumption within reasonable levels, and stay away from artificial colors and flavors. Take up a regular exercise routine; allow yourself to begin slowly and work your routine up if you are not used to exercising. Make sure all your personal care and hygiene products are made from natural substances with ingredients you can recognize. Do not use any products containing parabens or phthalates as these have been shown to be carcinogenic. Use natural products to clean your home and laundry.

Yes, this may seem like a drastic change in lifestyle, so I recommend that you being with just one thing and then every week add another change. It will be worth it to reduce the risk of developing a second cancer.

SUN SENSITIVITY

Sun sensitivity may show itself in many ways: Rash, hives, blisters, darkened blotches or increase susceptibility to sunburn are all signs of sun sensitivity. Some chemotherapy agents may cause your skin to be more sensitive to sunlight causing these reactions even if you have never had these reactions before. Associated chemotherapy agents include 5-fluorouracil, methotrexate, dacarbazine, vinblastine, docetaxel, doxorubicin, etoposide, and gemcitabine. You should also be aware that some other prescription medications besides chemotherapy agents may also cause sun sensitivity, such as certain antibiotics, antihistamines containing diphenhydramine, and certain acne treatments, among others. Talk to your prescribing doctors if you have any questions about the medications you are currently using.

The best way to handle sun sensitivity is to simply protect yourself from the sun's light: Use sunscreen,[75] wear long sleeves and wide brimmed hats, wear sunglasses, stay in the shade when possible, and be sure you use lip balm that contains sunscreen. If you do not have hair on your head you can opt for using sunscreen on your scalp, a wig, or a light cotton scarf. It is also wise to forgo tanning beds for the duration of your chemotherapy treatments. Do not undergo cosmetic skin treatments such as microdermabrasion, chemical peels, laser treatments or exfoliating facial scrubs. Be sure you are not using any personal care products containing alpha-hydroxy acids, beta-hydroxy acids, tretinoins, or benzoyl peroxide. It is also wise to avoid herbs, foods, and supplements which encourage sun sensitivity such as St. John's wort, angelica, arnica, celery, dill, fennel, figs, dong quai, rue, kava, parsley, yohimbe, lime peel and lemon peel.

---

75 If you are using any topical chemotherapy agents be sure to consult with your oncologist before applying sunscreen to the treatment area. Do not use products containing parabens or phthalates as these are known carcinogens.

WHITE BLOOD CELLS

Having a low number of white blood cells is known in the medical world as *leukopenia*. (*leuko* = white, *penia* = deficiency) and is a common side effect with some chemotherapy agents. Because white blood cells are vital to a functioning immune system a decrease in these cells usually results in an inability to fight off diseases and infections. Due to the high risk of infection patients with leukopenia should avoid crowded places in which one could easily catch cold, flu, or other communicable diseases. Stay away from people with any herpes infections including chicken pox and shingles. Make sure your foods are thoroughly cooked and that you do not eat any foods which are expired, old, or showing signs of spoilage (moldy spots, wilted spots, etc.)

Although there are some prescription medications known to reduce leukopenia there are none that can prevent it completely. Holistic methods are available to help boost white blood cell counts however these do take a little time to show results. For example, making sure you have an adequate intake of protein helps your body to form more cells in general, and this would include white blood cells. It should also be noted that vitamins B12 and B9 (folate) are necessary for forming new white blood cells, so speak to your doctor about whether you should supplement with these vitamins. You should also consult with your practitioner regarding the use of herbs and supplements such as astragalus, cat's claw, Chinese formula Bu Zhong Yi Qi, garlic, scaly wood mushroom, selenium, and zinc. Yogurt with active cultures has also been shown to help regulate white blood cell activity. Take note that anything which helps increase white blood cell counts has the potential to interfere with immune-modulating chemotherapy regimens. Be sure to discuss whether this type of supplementation is right for your therapeutic plan.

If you are dealing with any form of leukemia speak with your oncologist before using any products to boost white blood cell production. This is because leukemia is a cancer of the white blood cells, therefore you do not want to increase production during treatment, though with your doctor's advice it may be okay to use such products after treatment.

Chapter 6
HERBS, NUTRIENTS, AND SUPPLEMENTS

All items listed in this chapter are written the adult patient in mind as many of these have not been established as safe for children. When selecting a product only use those which are known to produce consistent, quality products. Independent testing has found companies whose products were mislabeled, contaminated with heavy metals, or were mixed with other substances not listed in the ingredients. Look for labels which have "USP",[76] "NSF International,"[77] "Consumer Lab," "USDA Organic" or "Green Screened" printed on them. Do not mix herbs or supplements without the advice of a competent practitioner as some substances may not work well together. Always consult with your prescribing physicians before starting a new herb or supplement to reduce risk of side effects or adverse interactions with your other medications.

ACETYL – L – CARNITINE:

Acetyl L-carnitine is an amino acid found in foods such as red meats, seafood, chicken and milk. However, since healthy kidneys can make acetyl L-carnitine vegans usually do not need supplementation. Some studies have shown that using supplements of this amino acid may help reduce some of the side effects caused by chemotherapy treatments. For example, it may help reduce the symptoms of nerve damage related to paclitaxel and cisplatin regimens,[78] and may help protect your heart and liver from damage caused by doxorubicin regimens.[79] [80] However, it should be noted that supplementation during treatment with taxanes showed an increase in neuropathy (nerve damage) after six months.[81] If you choose to use this supplement know that typical supplementation is usually 500 mg, three times per day. Generally speaking, up to 2,000 mg per day is considered safe. If your doctor decides you need more do not take more than 5,000 mg per day as it may cause digestive issues or rash. When taking it to protect your heart use it before you start your chemotherapy cycle *and* throughout your cycle of treatment. Along with the acetyl L-carnitine take up to 300 mg of co-enzyme Q10 (CoQ10) supplements to help your heart muscles produce more energy. *Precautions: Do not use supplements of this amino acid if you have an under-active thyroid. May induce seizures in patients with seizure disorders.*

---

76 USP = United States Pharmacopoeia

77 NSF = National Sanitation Foundation

78 *Acetyl-L-carnitine for the Treatment of Chemotherapy-Induced Peripheral Neuropathy* (De Grandis, 2007)

79 *L-Carnitine Prevents Doxorubicin-induced Apoptosis of Cardiac Myocytes: Role of Inhibition of Ceramide Generation.* (Andrieu-Abadie, 1999)

80 *Doxorubicin Toxicity can Be Ameliorated During Antioxidant L-Carnitine Supplementation.* (Alshabanah, 2010)

81 *Randomized Double-Blind Placebo-Controlled Trial of Acetyl-L-carnitine for the Prevention of Taxane-Induced Neuropathy in Women Undergoing Adjuvant Breast Cancer Therapy .*(Hershman, 2013)

ALOE:[82]

Aloe barbadensis/Aloe vera

This plant, also known as "Burn Plant", is famous for its skin-conditioning qualities. Its fleshy leaves contain an enzyme called bradykinase which relieves skin inflammation, polysaccharides and gibberellin which promote skin regeneration, and mucopolysaccharides which help keep moisture in the skin. Use of this plant during cancer treatment is supported by one case study in Brazil in which a cancer patient suffering from hand foot syndrome significantly improved after forty days of applying aloe gel to the skin lesions.[83] This well-known houseplant has also been shown to increase the effectiveness of the chemotherapy agents 5-fluorouracil and cyclophosphamide when used internally.[84] A typical dose is ¼ cup of aloe gel (60 ml) up to three times per day as tolerated. Do not drink juice made from whole aloe leaf because the inner portion of the leaf contains a strong laxative known as aloin. If you have a large, healthy plant already at home you can avoid the aloin simply by eating only the clear gel inside the leaves. Simply remove 4 tablespoons of gel (60 ml) and consume three times daily. Be sure you consume only the clear gel and no scrapings from inside the leaf skin. If, instead, you want to use the plant's gel for skin application be sure to speak to your oncologist and practitioners first if you are having any kind of skin-related treatments (radiation, heat therapy, essential oils, chemotherapeutic salves, etc.) as you do not want the gel to interfere with the effects of your treatments. *Precautions: Do not drink the juice if you have diarrhea or other bowel issues. Aloe may enhance immune resistance, so be sure to speak to your oncologist first if you are on any sort of immunotherapy or immuno-suppressants. Oral consumption of the gel may block the absorption of other oral medications taken at the same time. Some practitioners warn against using aloe concurrently with steroids, licorice root, or prescription diuretics. Always check with your practitioner before use, especially on broken skin or open sores.*

ALPHA-LIPOIC ACID:

Do not confuse alpha-lipoic acid with the similar sounding omega 3 fatty acid known as alpha-linolenic acid (which are both abbreviated as "ALA"). Alpha-lipoic acid is a water soluble and fat soluble antioxidant made within the body. Supplementation at 600mg per day in divided doses is commonly used for helping reduce the risk of neuropathy in patients being treated for myeloma. Because ALA is an anti-oxidant you should consult with your oncologist to be sure it will not diminish the effects of certain chemotherapy or radiation treatments you may be undergoing. Alpha-lipoic acid is also known to strengthen the effects of 5-fluorouracil and reduce the incidence of neuropathy during docetaxel-based regimens. One study investigating alpha-lipoic acid with docetaxel/cisplatin combination regimen used the

---

82 There is also another aloe variety, *Aloe arborescens*, which is said to have stronger healing properties than *Aloe barbadensis*. Because it is stronger I recommend using with professional guidance.

83 *[Hand-foot syndrome induced by chemotherapy: a case study]* (Simão, 2012, Original article in Portuguese)

84 **Scientific Basis for Ayurvedic Therapies**, p. 299, Edited by: Lakshmi Chandra Mishra, 2003

following doses with good results: 600mg of I.V. alpha-lipoic acid once weekly for 3-5 weeks followed with 1800mg twice daily by mouth until full recovery from neurological symptoms or up to 6 months, whichever came first. Out of the fourteen patients using this regimen eight experienced reduction in symptoms, taking an average of eight chemotherapy courses to start seeing results.[85] Studies also suggest that alpha-lipoic acid may reduce the side effects caused by cyclophosphamide[86] and lower the risk of hearing loss associated with cisplatin treatments in certain patients.[87] If, after consulting with your oncologist, you choose to supplement with alpha-lipoic acid, know that the common oral dosage is usually 300-600mg daily for four weeks. To reduce the risk of possible side effects from the supplement itself start with the lower dose and work your way up according to your tolerance level. *Precautions: One study using myeloma cells showed that alpha-lipoic acid may reduce the effectiveness of treatments using velcade. Because adding alpha-lipoic acid to your regimen may lower blood sugar levels and reduce levels of vitamin B1 (thiamine) I strongly advise patients to consult with their prescribing physicians before supplementing.*

AMERICAN GINSENG
Panax quinquefolius

Also known as Wisconsin ginseng; do not confuse with Asian ginseng (*panax ginseng*) or Siberian ginseng (*Eleutherococcus senticosus*). One double-blind pilot study involving 290 cancer patients observed that those who used American ginseng supplements tended to experience noticeably reduced cancer-related fatigue compared to patients who did not use the supplement.[88] This same researcher later performed a phase III study with 364 patients, observing that doses of 2,000mg American ginseng per day for 8 weeks seemed to be of most benefit on the average. This study also found that American ginseng worked better for patients who were receiving active cancer treatments vs. those who had already completed their treatments.[89] It is recommended that supplements contain at least 3% active ginsenosides for greatest effect. *Precautions: Take with food. May have estrogenic effect when taken as a methanol (alcohol) extract; use a water based extract instead. May act as a blood thinner. May interfere with your body's metabolism of certain other medications.*

APIGENIN:

This antioxidant bioflavonoid is found in plant sources such as apples, bacopa, cherries, grapes, rosemary, German chamomile, parsley, celery, basil, tea and wine;

85 *Amelioration of docetaxel/cisplatin induced polyneuropathy by α-lipoic acid* (Gedlicka, 2003)
86 *Effect of DL-alpha-lipoic Acid on Cyclophosphamide Induced Lysosomal Changes in Oxidative Cardiotoxicity.* (Mythili, 2007)
87 *Alpha-lipoic Acid Protects Against Cisplatin-induced Ototoxicity via the Regulation of MAPKs and Proinflammatory Cytokines.* (Kim, 2014)
88 *Pilot study of Panax quinquefolius (American ginseng) to improve cancer-related fatigue: a randomized, double-blind, dose-finding evaluation: NCCTG trial N03CA* (Barton, 2010)
89 *Wisconsin Ginseng (Panax quinquefolius) to Improve Cancer-Related Fatigue: A Randomized, Double-Blind Trial, N07C2.* (Barton, 2013)

however it can also be bought as a commercial nutritional supplement. Apigenin inhibits the body's production of aromatase, an enzyme used in the production of estrogen, therefore, this substance may be useful for patients who are fighting an estrogen-fueled cancer. In vitro studies have also shown apigenin to activate the p53 gene,[90] the gene which induces cell suicide in many types of cancerous cells and hinders the process of blood vessel formation in tumors through inhibition of the VEGF protein.[91] Other studies have observed that apigenin enhances the anti-cancer effect of paclitaxel agents[92] as well as help reduce anxiety. Dosage range is 3-10mg of apigenin per kilogram of body weight (2-5mg per pound). Higher doses may cause sedation and is not recommended without the advice of your doctor or practitioner. *Precautions: Because many natural sources of apigenin also contain large amounts of antioxidants be sure your chemotherapy regimen does not require avoidance of antioxidants before you start increasing your dietary intake of this substance.*

ARNICA
Arnica montana

This herb is also known as wolfsbane, leopard's bane, mountain arnica, and mountain tobacco. This herb is well-known for its skin healing properties and therefore many like to use it as an oral rinse for mouth sores. However arnica, which is classified as an unsafe herb by the FDA, is highly toxic if swallowed. Therefore I do not recommend use as a full-strength mouth rinse. Instead you should use homeopathic arnica preparations (with professional guidance) as these are prepared at much safer dilutions. Never use on children or babies. Arnica may be applied to the skin, however you must be sure that any arnica preparations you use will not interfere with any topical treatments you may be undergoing. This may include topical chemotherapy agents, other herbal skin treatments, local heat therapy, local light therapy, etc. *Precautions: Do not use if you are allergic to plants in the ragweed family. Do not use more than recommended amounts; this includes use as a topical skin treatment.*

ASIAN GINSENG:
Panax ginseng

Also known as Chinese ginseng, Korean ginseng, and red ginseng. Do not confuse this with American ginseng (*Panax quinquefolius*) or Siberian ginseng (*Eleutherococcus senticosus*). Asian ginseng contains ginsenosides, substances which are known to be adaptogenic, i.e. helps the body cope with stress and fatigue. One small study supplied 30 patients with 800mg Asian ginseng for 29 days, showing marked improvement in fatigue symptoms among 87% of the patients by the fifteenth day.[93] Studies have also shown that ginsenoside-Rg3 can weaken chemo-resistance

---

90 *Evidence for Activation of Mutated p53 by Apigenin in Human Pancreatic Cancer* (King, 2012)

91 *[Effect and Mechanism of Apigenin on VEGF Expression in Human Breast Cancer Cells* (X. Y. Jin, 2007) (translated from an article originally written in Chinese)

92 *Synergistic Effects of Apigenin and Paclitaxel on Apoptosis of Cancer Cells* (Yimiao Xu, 2012)

93 *High-Dose Asian Ginseng (Panax Ginseng) for Cancer-Related Fatigue: A Preliminary Report* (Yennurajalingam,, 2015)

57

cancer cells[94] and protect healthy cells from damage caused by cyclophosphamide treatments.[95] Another study showed that ginsenoside Rh2 can inhibit the growth of melanoma and ovarian cancer cells[96] as well as reduce chemo-resistance in breast cancer cells.[97] In vitro and in vivo studies have shown some other ginsenosides can inhibit the growth of prostate cancer and can be safely combined with docetaxel and gemcitabine.[98] One particular review of studies observed that Asian ginseng enhances the action of chemotherapy agents such as 5-fluorouracil, irinotecan, mitomycin-C, docetaxel, doxorubicin, and cisplatin, inhibits the growth of colon cancer cells, and certain melanoma cells, reduces cisplatin-induced kidney damage, and that a ginsenoside-Rg3 can inhibit tumor blood vessel formation, especially when used with gemcitabine or cyclophosphamide. This review also noted that the combination of Asian ginseng with various chemotherapy agents reduced side effects such as nausea, diaphragm muscle damage caused by doxorubicin, liver damage, and kidney damage.[99] *Precautions: Asian ginseng may work against immunosuppressive therapies. May cause insomnia, headache, menstrual problems, dizziness, changes in blood pressure, heart rhythm changes, worsen psychiatric disorders, lower blood sugar levels, and may thin the blood. Interacts with several medications and herbs, so use under close supervision. May have estrogenic effect when extracted with methanol (alcohol); use water extracted preparations instead if you have an estrogen-fueled cancer. Do not use if you've had an organ transplant at it may encourage organ rejection. May interact with alcohol, caffeine, and diuretics. May interfere with CYP substrates (see chapter 7 of this book).*

ASTRAGALUS:
Astragalus membranaceus/ A. propinquus / A. penduliflorus

This is a popular herb known in Traditional Chinese Medicine as Huang Qi. Astragalus extracts have been effective in reducing inflammation and enhancing blood cell counts as well as helping patients reduce cancer-related fatigue.[100] This herb has also been observed to be protective of the heart and liver from the effects of chemotherapy-induced damages[101] [102] while it also induces cell death in liver cancer

94 *Selective Toxicity of Ginsenoside-Rg3 on Multidrug resistant Cells by Membrane Fluidity Modulation.* (Kwon, 2008)

95 *Protective Effects of Ginsenoside-Rg3 Against Cyclophosphamide-induced DNA Damage and Cell Apoptosis in Mice.* (Zhang, 2008)

96 *Inhibitory Effects of Ginsenoside-Rh2 on Tumor Growth in Nude Mice Bearing Human Ovarian Cancer Cells.* (Nakata, 1998).

97 *Ginsenoside Rh2 Differentially Mediates MicrRNA Expression to Prevent Chemoresistance of Breast Cancer* (Wen, 2015)

98 *Experimental Therapy of Prostate Cancer with Novel Natural Product Anti-cancer Ginsenosides.* (Wang, 2008)

99 *Ginseng and Anticancer Drug Combination to Improve Cancer Chemotherapy: A Critical Review.* (Shihong Chen, 2014)

100 *A novel infusible botanically-derived drug, PG2, for cancer-related fatigue: a phase II double-blind, randomized placebo-controlled study* (H. W. Chen, 2012)

101 *Astragalus Polysaccharide Suppresses Doxorubicin-induced Cardiotoxicity by Regulating the PI3k/Akt and p38MAPK Pathways* (Yuan Cao, 2014)

102 *Protective Effect of Astragalus polysaccharides on Liver Injury Induced by Several Different*

cells,[103] and colon cancer cells.[104] Another study observed that using astragalus along with vinblastine slows colon cancer by inhibiting tumor blood vessel formation.[105] Combining astragalus with Asian ginseng (*panax ginseng*) may increase the survival of lung cancer patients being treated with methotrexate and vincristine. In mouse models astragalus was shown to enhance the action of 5-fluorouracil in mice with stomach tumors[106] while another study showed that it enhances the effects of pterosilbene against melanomas.[107] Other studies have shown that using astragalus with platinum-based chemotherapy may increase patient survival rate and improves tumor response.[108] There are hundreds of scientific studies that have been performed with astragalus too numerous to mention in this book, but the main point is that astragalus can be a potent warrior in your fight against cancer. Typical dosage of astragalus is as follows: Combine 1 tsp. (5ml) astragalus tincture with 1 tsp. (5ml) ginseng tincture in ¼ cup of water (60ml) and consume three times daily. May increase the tinctures to 4 tsp. each per dose as needed. If using capsules the typical dosage is one 250mg – 500mg capsule three to four times daily. [109] or make a tea with 7ml of powdered root (1 ½ tsp.) to 12 ounces of boiling water three times daily, or 20-60 drops of tincture (30% ethanol) three times daily. *Precautions: Astragalus can increase urination and, as a result, might affect the elimination of the drug lithium leading to serious side effects. Astragalus may also affect blood sugar levels and blood pressure. This herb is known to thin the blood, please use caution if you are on prescribed anticoagulants. This herb has antioxidant activity, estrogenic properties, and immune-stimulating properties which may interfere with the actions of certain chemotherapy treatments. Be sure to speak to your oncologist before using astragalus with your treatment plan.*

BACOPA:

Bacopa monnieri

This Ayurvedic herb is also known as brahmi, do not confuse with the herb gotu kola (*Centella asiatica*) which also goes by the name of brahmi. Clinical trials have shown bacopa to significantly enhance memory retention in test subjects[110] as well as enhance the mental functioning of the elderly.[111] It has been shown to have

Chemotherapeutics in Mice. (Wen Liu, 2014)

103 *Astragalus polysaccharide induces the apoptosis of human hepatocellular carcinoma cells by decreasing the expression of Notch1.* (Huang, 2016)

104 *Astragalus saponins induce growth inhibition and apoptosis in human colon cancer cells and tumor xenograft.* (Tin, 2007)

105 *Combined therapeutic effects of vinblastine and Astragalus saponins in human colon cancer cells and tumor xenograft via inhibition of tumor growth and proangiogenic factors.* (Auyeung, 2014)

106 *Effect of 5-fluorouracil in combination with Astragalus membranaceus on amino acid metabolism in mice model of gastric carcinoma* (Z. X. Zhang, 2006)

107 *Enhanced antitumor efficacy with combined administration of astragalus and pterostilbene for melanoma* (X. Y. Huang, 2015)

108 *Astragalus-based Chinese herbs and platinum-based chemotherapy for advanced non-small-cell lung cancer: meta-analysis of randomized trials* (McCulloch, 2006)

109 Standardized to 0.4% 4-hydroxy-3-methoxy isoflavone 7-sug

110 *Chronic Effects of Brahmi (Bacopa monnieri) on Human Memory.* (Roodenrys, 2002)

111 *Effects of a standardized Bacopa monnieri extract on cognitive performance, anxiety, and*

anti-anxiety action similar to the prescription medication lorazepam[112] and has a painkilling effect comparable to diclofenac. It also inhibits morphine tolerance and enhances the painkilling effects of opiate medications. Long term use of bacopa does not result in tolerance to the herb.[113] Other research with mouse models have shown this herb to also have anti-depressant activity.[114] Dosage: Take 300mg of bacopa extract daily; oftentimes takes up to twelve weeks to reach full effect. Make sure the supplement has 55% bacoside compounds. To use the whole herb powder, take 750 – 1,500 mg of the powder daily. *Precautions: May slow the heart rate, cause constipation, or increase fluid formation in the lungs or urinary bladder. Do not use if you have thyroid problems. Constituents are fat soluble, therefore take with food containing healthy fats. May reduce male fertility during use. May slow down heart rate. Do not use if you have problems with intestinal blockage. May worsen ulcers. May worsen emphysema or asthma. Do not use if you have urinary obstructions.*

BAIKAL SKULLCAP :
Scutellaria baikalensis

This herb is also known as Chinese skullcap; do not confuse with American skullcap (*Scutellaria lateriflora*) or barbed skullcap (*Scutellaria barbata*). Baikal skullcap is also known as "goldenroot"; do not confuse this with goldenthread (*Coptis trifolia*), goldenseal (*Hydrastis canadensis*) or roseroot (*Rhodiola Rosea* which is also known as goldenroot). Studies have shown that baikal skullcap can cause cell death in human pancreatic cancer cells[115] and inhibit growth in several different cancer cells lines including squamous cell, prostate, liver, colon, and hormone-positive breast cancers.[116] It also contains a compound called *baikalein*, which is known to reduce heart damage caused by doxorubicin treatments[117] and enhance the action of the chemotherapy agent paclitaxel. [118] Another compound in this herb known as *baikalin*, when taken orally, can be converted in the intestines into baikalein, which inhibits the growth of colorectal cancer cells.[119] Both baikalein and baikalin have the ability to cross the blood-brain barrier and thus it has also been studied as a potential therapy against brain tumors. Studies have shown that use of baikal skullcap enhances the effects of the chemotherapy agent carmustine against glioblastoma brain cancers (it

depression in the elderly: a randomized, double-blind, placebo-controlled trial. (Calabrese, 2008)

112 *Anxiolytic activity of a standardized extract of Bacopa monniera: an experimental study.* (Bhattacharya, 1998)

113 *Preclinical Profile of Bacopasides from Bacopa monnieri (BM) as an Emerging Class of Therapeutics for Management of Chronic Pains.* (Rauf, 2013)

114 *Antidepressant-like effects of methanolic extract of Bacopa monniera in mice.* (Mannan, 2015)

115 *baikalein, a Component of Scutellaria baikalensis, Induces Apoptosis by Mcl-1 Down-regulation in Human Pancreatic Cancer Cells.* (Takahashi, 2011)

116 *Anticancer Activity of Scutellaria baikalensis and its Potential Mechanism.* (F. Ye, 2002)

117 *baikalein Protects Against Doxorubicin-induced Cardiotoxicity by Attenuation of Mitochondrial Oxidant Injury and JNK Activation.* (Chang, 2011)

118 *A Combination Therapy with baikalein and Taxol Promotes Mitochondria-Mediated Cell Apoptosis: Involving in Akt/β-Catenin Signaling Pathway.* (Pan, 2016)

119 *Colon cancer chemopreventive effects of baikalein, an active enteric microbiome metabolite from baikalin.* (Wang, 2015)

may also be used as supporting therapy along with other brain cancer agents).[120]   At the time of this writing there is no standard dosage for *S. baikalensis*. However, a commonly used dose for oral administration is between 5-15 grams of powdered root steeped in 1 cup (240ml) of boiling water to make a tea. *Precautions: Buy from a reputable source as some products may contain germander – a plant which may cause liver damage. May thin the blood. May affect cholesterol lowering drugs. Do not use with products containing dextromethorphan. May increase the activity of T-cells (an immune system component). May interact with alcohol or other sedatives to cause excessive drowsiness. Do not use if you are taking medications for diabetes or are on lithium. May have estrogenic effect; seek professional advice if you are battling an estrogen-fueled cancer. May lower blood pressure. Consult with your physician first if you have had an organ transplant. Consult with your physician if you have problems with your stomach, liver, kidneys, or spleen.*

BAKING SODA
Sodium bicarbonate

Some chemotherapy agents may cause mouth sores which can make oral hygiene difficult because toothpastes and mouthwashes can irritate the open sores. Instead of using commercial products you should use plain baking soda to clean your teeth sometimes. Not only is baking soda an excellent oral cleanser, but it is very alkali, which means it will neutralize any acids in your mouth that would further irritate your sores. Alternatively you may mix 1 tsp. Of baking soda in ½ cup of plain water and use as a mouth rinse. Simply sprinkle a small amount of baking soda onto your wet toothbrush bristles and brush your teeth like usual. Baking soda is also useful to counteract heartburn because it neutralizes the acid. Simply mix 1 tsp (15ml) of baking soda in 1 cup (240ml) of water, drink the entire mixture. *Precautions: Using baking soda on your teeth more than two or three times per week may cause damage to your tooth enamel. Baking soda cleans but does not kill germs; rinse with a gentle, alcohol-free mouthwash after brushing. Do not use baking soda on braces or retainers. Baking soda is high in sodium, therefore do not use for heartburn more than two times per day.*

BERBERINE:

Although this can be found as a natural supplement in the vitamin aisle this yellow alkaloid is naturally present in abundance within herbs such as barberry (*Berberis vulgaris*), goldenthread (*Coptis chinensis*), goldenseal (*Hydrastis canadensis*),[121] Oregon grape (*Mahonia aquifolium*), and tree turmeric (*Berberis aristata*).[122] In vitro studies have shown berberine to be effective against various cancers through interruption of the cancer cells' abilities to reproduce and induction of cancer cell death. Several hundred published papers confirm that berberine is effective against

---

120 *Anticancer activity of extracts derived from the mature roots of Scutellaria baikalensis on human malignant brain tumor cells.* (Scheck, 2006)

121 *H. canadensis* contains more berberine than its relative *c. chinensis* on this list.

122 Do not confuse tree turmeric with Javanese turmeric (*curcuma xanthorrhiza*) or regular turmeric (*curcuma longa*). These are each different herbs.

brain tumors and a wide range of other cancers. In vitro studies have found that when berberine and curcumin (a substance in the spice turmeric, a.k.a. *Curcuma longa*) are combined they have synergistic effect against ER+ and triple negative breast cancer cells which works better than either substance alone.[123] One study observed that the use of goldenthread root (*Coptidis rhizoma*) inhibits the growth of esophageal cancers.[124] One review of studies found that cancer cell types sensitive to berberine include leukemia, liver, lung, stomach, colon, skin, oral, esophagus, brain, bone, breast and hormone-fueled cells. Berberine usually inhibits cancer through cell death but can also slow down cancer through other methods. The review also noted that berberine has shown synergistic effect with chemotherapy agents fighting ER+ breast cancers, as well as arsenic trioxide.[125] Other studies have shown berberine to re-sensitize cancer cells to chemotherapy agents such as 5-fluorouracil,[126] and cisplatin,[127] among others. Typical dosage of berberine supplement is 500 – 2,000 mg daily in divided doses (do not take more than 500mg at a time) with meals. Dosing is dependent upon your overall health; be sure to consult with a competent practitioner. *Precautions: Is known to reduce blood sugar. May lower blood pressure. High doses may cause digestive issues and diarrhea. Too much berberine may decrease muscle mass. Herbs and supplements containing berberine may prolong Qtc in patients with certain types of heart disease. May cause jaundice in those with liver problems.*

BERGAMOT FRUIT:
Citrus Bergamia

Do not confuse with the herb named "bergamot" (*Monarda didyma*). Bergamot is a citrus fruit used in foods such as Earl Grey Tea, Turkish delight, and some marmalades. The oil is extracted from the peel and can be used medicinally. Researchers have found that bergamot juice extract reduced the growth of colorectal cancers by inducing cell death when taken in low concentrations, and causing DNA damage in cancer cells, thus killing them, in high concentrations.[128] Another study showed that applying bergamot oil to skin and then treating the area with ultraviolet light is effective against skin fungal infections. Studies have shown that substances in the essential oil of bergamot used in aromatherapy are as effective at reducing anxiety as diazepam,[129] reduces anxiety in pre-operative patients,[130] and reduces work related

---

123 *Synergistic Chemopreventive Effects of Curcumin and Berberine on Human Breast Cancer Cells Through Induction of Apoptosis and Autophagic Cell Death.* (Wang, 2016)

124 *Inhibitory effect of Coptidis Rhizoma and berberine on the proliferation of human esophageal cancer cell lines.* (Iizuka, 2000)

125 *Berberine and Coptidis Rhizoma as novel antineoplastic agents: a review of traditional use and biomedical investigations.* (Jun Tang, 2009)

126 *Berberine Reverses the Chemoresistance of Breast Cancer to 5- Fluorouracil by Downregulating Metadherin* (Kong 2012)

127 *Berberine sensitizes ovarian cancer cells to cisplatin through miR-21/PDCD4 axis* (Liu, 2013)

128 *Bergamot Juice Extract Inhibits Proliferation by Inducing Apoptosis in Human Colon Cancer Cells.* (Giuseppa, 2014)

129 *Acute Effects of Bergamot Oil on Anxiety-related Behaviour and Corticosterone Level in Rats.* (Saiyudthong, 2011)

130 *The Anxiolytic Effect of Aromatherapy on Patients Awaiting Ambulatory Surgery: A Randomized*

stress. It has also been successfully used as an appetite stimulant. As of this writing there are no standard doses set for bergamot, however some practitioners may recommend up to four 500mg capsules of bergamot oil per day for internal use. *Precautions: Bergamot may lower blood sugar or interfere with blood sugar during surgery, therefore do not use it for two weeks before a surgical procedure. Bergamot oil may cause increased sun sensitivity. Do not use with medications which are also contraindicated for grapefruit.*

BERRIES:

One study showed that cranberry was effective for decreasing heart damage in animal models which were given doxorubicin.[131] Because bilberries and blueberries are so closely related to cranberries it is thought that these may also have a similar effect. Although studies are promising in animal models, as of this writing human studies have not been confirmed. If you choose to increase your berry consumption based on these animal studies please note that the fresher the berries the better, as excessive processing of the fruit tends to destroy therapeutic properties. I highly recommend growing your own when possible. *Precautions: Berries tend to be high in antioxidants. Be sure the antioxidant activity will not reduce the efficacy of your current chemotherapy treatments.*

β-ELEMENE, a.k.a. BETA -ELEMENE:

This is a substance derived from the plants zedoary (*Rhizoma zedoariae*) and wild turmeric (*Curcuma aromatica*), as well as celery, ginger, and mint. It is not sold as a dietary supplement. Research has shown this substance to have broad-spectrum anti-tumor properties against several types of cancer[132] and has been used to successfully reverse multiple drug resistance in cancer treatments.[133] This substance has also been known to increase the effectiveness of radiation treatments as well as the chemotherapy medications cisplatin and taxanes. One review of studies showed that the use of β-elemene in patients with non-small cell lung cancer showed significant increases in survival time, quality of life, and decreased tumor activity in patients who used β-elemene in comparison with patients who did not.[134] Another study showed β-elemene to inhibit the growth and metastasis of melanoma through inhibition of tumor blood vessel formation.[135] This substance can also cross the blood-brain barrier and has been shown to inhibit the proliferation of human glioblastoma cells.[136] *Precautions: Do not use Zedoary if you are on blood thinners. As for wild*

Controlled Trial. (Ni, 2013)

131 *Cranberry (Vaccinium macrocarpon) Protects Against Doxorubicin-Induced Cardiotoxicity in Rats* (Elberry, 2010)

132 *Antineoplastic Effect of Beta-elemene on Prostate Cancer Cells and Other Types of Solid Tumor Cells.* (Li, 2010)

133 *The reversal of antineoplastic drug resistance in cancer cells by β-elemene* Guan-Nan (Zhang, 2015)

134 *Systematic Review of β-elemene Injection as Adjunctive Treatment for Lung Cancer.* (Wang, 2012)

135 *Beta-elemene Inhibits Melanoma Growth and Metastasis Via Suppressing Vascular Endothelial Growth Factor-mediated Angiogenesis.* (Chen, 2011)

136 *B-elemene Inhibits Proliferation of Human Glioblastoma Cells Through the Activation of Glia*

turmeric it is closely related to culinary turmeric. Due to turmeric's variability on how it works with cancer I strongly advise you not to use it without professional guidance. Because β-elemene can enhance the effects of chemotherapy medications use this only under the tandem guidance of your oncologist and practitioner in order to avoid potential toxic side effects from your chemotherapy treatments.

BITTER GREENS:

Bitter greens include leafy vegetables such as arugula, kale, collards, radicchio, watercress, dandelion greens, and endive. Beyond adding healthy vitamins, minerals, and fiber to your diet bitter greens also stimulate your digestive juices and enzymes thereby stimulating your appetite. You can either eat the greens or drink the juice made from the greens at least one-half hour before meals to help stimulate your appetite.

BLACK CUMIN
Nigella Sativa,/ Nigella cretica

Black cumin seed, also known as black seed, is well-known for its strong effects against cancer including both solid tumors and leukemia. In vivo studies have shown that when black cumin is combined with German Chamomile (*Matricaria chamomilla*) they work together to protect the kidneys from the chemotoxic effects of cisplatin.[137] Black cumin contains a substance called thymoquinone which is known to be effective against cancer. Thymoquinone has been shown to be protective against the effects of ifosfamide,[138] and doxorubicin-induced heart damage[139] without reducing the agents' effects (the latter study used an oral dose of 8mg thymoquinone per kg of weight [4mg per pound] daily). It also helps boost the efficacy of doxorubicin primarily through cell death.[140] Another study observed thymoquinone also inhibits the progression of tumor blood vessel formation and the growth of tumors through inhibition of the VEGF protein necessary for angiogenesis.[141] In yet another study it was observed that thymoquinone significantly increased the tumor-killing properties of the agents gemcitabine and oxaliplatin by at least three fold.[142] Black cumin seed tends to work best with cancers in stages I and II, especially when combined with 4-5 garlic cloves each day. Be sure to crush the raw garlic cloves and let sit for ten minutes before consuming to allow the constituents in the garlic to

---

Maturation Factor Beta and Induces Sensitization to Cisplatin. (Zhu, 2011)

137 *Nephroprotective Effect of Nigella Sativa and Matricaria Chamomilla in Cisplatin Induced Renal Injury* (Salama, 2011)

138 *Thymoquinone attenuates ifosfamide-induced Fanconi syndrome in rats and enhances its antitumor activity in mice.* (Badary, 1999)

139 *Thymoquinone protects against doxorubicin-induced cardiotoxicity without compromising its antitumor activity..* (al-Shabanah, 1998).

140 *Combinatorial Effects of Thymoquinone on the Anti-cancer Activity of Doxorubicin.* (Effenberger-Neidnicht, 2011)

141 *Thymoquinone inhibits tumor angiogenesis and tumor growth through suppressing AKT and extracellular signal-regulated kinase signaling pathways.* (Yi, 2008)

142 *Antitumor activity of gemcitabine and oxaliplatin is augmented by thymoquinone in pancreatic cancer.* (Banerjee, 2009)

synthesize the necessary healing compounds within itself first. To use whole black cumin seed: Grind or pound the seeds into powder as whole seed will simply pass through your system and waste all benefits. Put the powder into medicinal capsules or drink with water. Be very careful that you do not take more than 500mg of black seed powder daily. Take this on a empty stomach. Some practitioners will tell you to heat the seeds before consumption, however if you do this it will reduce their effectiveness against cancer.[143] To use the oil: Start with 1 teaspoon (5ml) daily; work your way up to 3 teaspoons (15ml) daily. Do not take more than this without speaking with your doctor first. Take this on an empty stomach. To use capsules: Generally speaking, two capsules of oil are equal to 1 teaspoon. Therefore, start with only two capsules daily and work your way up to six capsules daily. Take on an empty stomach. *Precautions: Black cumin may lower blood sugar, lower blood pressure, and slow your blood clotting response. Discontinue use at least two weeks before any surgery. May change white blood cells counts. More than 25g per day may cause liver damage. May cause skin allergy in some people. Black cumin seed and its oil is anti-oxidant therefore check with your oncologist to be sure this will not affect your chemotherapy agents*

BLACK PEPPER / PIPERINE:

Piperine is found primarily in black peppercorns (*Piper nigrum*) and in lower amounts in long peppers (*Piper longum*). This is the substance that gives black peppercorns their spicy flavor and pungent aroma. In vitro studies have observed that piperine reverses multi-drug resistance in breast cancers,[144] and inhibits the growth of colon cancer,[145] and prostate cancer,[146] Aromatherapeutically, inhalation of essential oil of black pepper has also been shown to significantly increase epinephrine levels in the system giving an invigorating response to counteract fatigue, though it is not recommended if you also experience bouts of anxiety. *Precautions: Normal dietary amounts of black pepper are generally safe. Do not overuse supplements. Piperine interacts with lithium and medications which are changed by the liver. Do not use pure or concentrated piperine without the strict oversight of a physician. Piperine interacts with CYP3A4 substrates (see chapter 7 of this book); check to be sure it is compatible with your other medications or chemotherapy agents.*

BLUSHWOOD BERRIES:

Fontainea picrosperma

These tropical fruits grow only in certain parts of Australia and have been found to contain a substance known a EBC-46 in their seeds, a compound which kills

---

143 *Volatile compounds of black cumin seeds (Nigella sativa L.) from microwave-heating and conventional roasting.* (Kiralan, 2012)

144 *Piperine, a piperidine alkaloid from Piper nigrum re-sensitizes P-gp, MRP1 and BCRP dependent multidrug resistant cancer cells* (Li, 2011)

145 *Piperine, an alkaloid from black pepper, inhibits growth of human colon cancer cells via G1 arrest and apoptosis triggered by endoplasmic reticulum stress.*(Yaffe, 2015)

146 *Piperine, a Bioactive Component of Pepper Spice Exerts Therapeutic Effects on Androgen Dependent and Androgen Independent Prostate Cancer Cells* (Samykutty, 2013)

cancer cells by targeting a protein called kinase-C.[147] Tests on animals such as dogs, cats, and horses have shown EBC-46 to have tremendous promise in fighting various types of cancers. Human trials, performed by injecting EBC-46 directly into solid tumors have shown destruction of the tumors withing 48 hours of treatment. According to Dr. Glen Boyle, of the Queensland Institute of Medical Research "*In most cases the single injection treatment caused the loss of viability of cancer cells within four hours, and ultimately destroyed the tumors... In more than 70% of pre-clinical cases, the response and cure was long-term and enduring, with very little relapse over a period of twelve months*." He went on to note that this treatment may not be effective for metastatic cancers. Although blushwood berries are an extremely promising ally against cancer there are two major obstacles to mass production of the agent: Not only are they very specific in their growing conditions, but it also takes three weeks to finish the extraction process of EBC-46. Researchers hope to find a way to synthesize EBC-46 to make it more widely available to patients. At this time the treatment is being given only by direct injection into solid tumors. *Precautions: The berries are extremely toxic; do not attempt to make home-made cancer treatments with this fruit.*

BOSWELLIA:
Boswellia serrata

Also known as "Indian frankincense," do not confuse with Norwegian frankincense (*Albies excelsa*). Boswellia is well-known for its anti-inflammatory properties[148] due to substances contained within which are similar to steroids. It is especially effective in reducing the production of Tumor Necrosis Factor-A (TNF-Alpha), an inflammatory cytokine. One study showed that boswellia significantly reduced formation of blood vessels in prostate cancer tumors by suppressing the VEGF proteins.[149] Because steroid medications used for reducing swelling and inflammation oftentimes interfere with the effects of chemotherapy agents such as camptothecin (especially with brain cancers) the anti-inflammatory properties of boswellia can be a viable alternative. Not only does boswellia have the ability to cross the blood-brain barrier, but its components have been shown to be toxic to glioma cancer cells.[150] [151] In Europe boswellia is commonly used for treating peri-tumoral edema in brain cancer patients.[152] One case study reported on a HER2+ breast cancer patient who developed metastasis to the brain with several inoperable tumors. The report states that after ten weeks of treatment with 800mg. of boswellia three times daily along with the chemotherapy agent capecitabine all signs of brain metastasis

---

147 *Intra-lesional Injection of the Novel PKC Activator EBC-46 Rapidly Ablates Tumors in Mouse Models.* (Boyle, 2014)

148 *Boswellia Serrata, A Potential Anti-inflammatory Agent: An Overview.* (Siddiqui, 2011)

149 *Acetyl-11-keto-beta – boswellic acid Inhibits Prostate Tumor Growth by Suppressing Vascular Endothelial Growth Factor Receptor 2- mediated Angiogenesis* (Pang, 2009)

150 *Boswellic Acids ad Malignant Glioma: Induction of Apoptosis but no Modulation of Drug Sensitivity* (Glaser, 1999)

151 *Boswellic Acids Inhibit Glioma Growth; A New Treatment Option?* (Winking, 2000)

152 *Determination of Boswellic Acids in Brain and Plasma by High-performance Liquid Chromatography/Tandem Mass Spectrometry* (Reising, 2005)

had disappeared. At the time of the report the patient survived over four years (whereas the average life expectancy for her condition should have been 3-5 *months*).[153] Other studies have observed that boswellic acids in the herb can reduce the growth of multiple myeloma[154] and other leukemia cells lines[155] as well as the growth of glioma brain cancers.[156] Boswellia should be given orally every six hours to maintain blood plasma levels of the substance. Administration with a high fat meal significantly increases the body's absorption of the substance. Typical dosage is 800mg extract, standardized to 65% boswellic acids, three times daily. Can take up to 1,200 mg three times daily if needed. May also take in tablet or capsule form. *Precautions: Is a known blood thickener. Consult with your prescribing physicians if you are already on a topoisomerase inhibitor such as irinotecan because this is also an inhibitor. May cause mild stomach upset. If on long-term, high dose therapy with boswellia do not suddenly stop as it may cause rebound effects such as tumoral edema. May cause digestive issues, rash, or allergic reactions. Do not take for longer than six months.*

BRASSICA / CRUCIFEROUS VEGETABLES:

Brassicas, a.k.a. cruciferous vegetables[157] contain sulforaphane, a known anti-cancer substance. Because sulforaphane is able to cross the blood-brain barrier it has been studied for use in destroying brain cancers. One study found that combining sulforaphane with the antioxidant resveratrol[158] helps induce cell death in human glioma cells in vitro.[159] Another study, using only sulforaphane, found that giving mice injections of sulforaphane for three weeks significantly reduced the size of glioma tumors.[160] Another study observed that sulforaphane inhibited glioblastoma brain cancers from migrating and invading[161] and yet another study showed sulforaphane to induce cell death in medulloblastoma cells.[162] Other studies also show sulforaphane to act against other types of brain cancer cells such as acoustic neuroma,

---

153 *A lipoxygenase inhibitor in breast cancer brain metastases.* (Flavin, 2007)

154 *Boswellic Acid Blocks Sigal Transducers and Activators of Transcription 3 Signaling Proliferation and Survival of Multiple Myeloma via the Protein Tyrosine Phosphatase SHP-1* (Kunnumakkara, 2009)

155 *Boswellic Acid Acetate Induces Differentiation and Apoptosis in Leukemia Cell Lines* (Jing, 1999)

156 *Boswellic Acids Inhibit Glioma Growth: a New Option?* (Winking, 2000)

157 Brassica vegetables include: Arugula, bok choy, cauliflower, all cabbages, collard greens, broccoli, broccoli rabe, Brussels sprouts, daikon, horseradish, kale, kohlrabi, komatsuna, mizuna, mustard greens, radishes, romanesco, rutabaga, tatsoi, turnips, turnip greens, wasabi, and watercress

158 *Natural sources of resveratrol include peanut skins, pistachios, red grapes, red wine, cranberries, and dark natural process cocoa.*

159 *Combination Treatment with Resveratrol and Sulforaphane Induces Apoptosis in Human U251 Glioma Cells.* (Hao Jiang,, 2010)

160 *Effects of Sulforaphane on Growth Inhibition in Human Brain Malignant Glioma GBM 8401 Cells by Means of Mitochondrial-and MEK/ERK-mediated Apoptosis Pathway.* (T. Y. Huang, 2012)

161 *Sulforaphane Inhibits Invasion via Activating ERK 1/ 2 Signaling in Human Glioblastoma U87MG and U373MG Cells* (Li, 2014)

162 *Induction of Medulloblastoma Cell Apoptosis by Sulforaphane, a Dietary Anticarcinogen from Brassica Vegetables* (Gingras, 2004)

astrocytoma, meningioma, and others. Aside from brain cancer sulforaphane has shown potential against other forms of human cancer cells such as breast, colon, ovarian, pancreatic, and prostate cancers. Sulforaphane is water soluble and heat sensitive, therefore it is better to eat your brassica vegetables very lightly cooked; do not boil them, or better yet, eat them raw. The only exceptions to using them raw are broccoli and broccoli sprouts: Broccoli and its sprouts contain a protein which binds the sulforaphane. Lightly heating the broccoli or the sprouts allows the protein to break down enough to release the sulforaphane. Therefore these should be steamed for only 2 minutes or microwaved (900W oven) for only 45 seconds (Broccoli and broccoli sprouts tend to be the best sources of sulforaphane).[163] Some sources state sulforaphane supplements give a more therapeutic dose than through diet alone. If you opt to take sulforaphane supplements be sure the supplements contain sulforaphane glucosinolate (SGS) that is obtained from broccoli or broccoli sprouts, not from the *seeds* of the plant. At the time of this writing there is no known optimal supplemental dose for sulforaphane. *Precautions: Sulfur compounds in brassica vegetables can interfere with thyroid function; therefore consult with your physician before increasing intake of brassicas or related supplements if you have thyroid problems. Do not take at the same time you take other medications to avoid interactions; take your doses at least two hours before or after.*

BROMELAIN:

This is an enzyme naturally present in pineapples and can also be bought as a commercial supplement. Although it is normally thought of as a substance to help with digestion and constipation it can also reduce inflammation thereby reducing pain, including post-surgical pain. In vitro and in vivo studies have also shown that this enzyme can inhibit cancer growth and increase cancer cell death.[164] Because the high temperatures involved in canning pineapple destroys bromelain it is best that you use only fresh pineapple or commercially prepared supplements for therapeutic purposes. The enzyme is easily absorbed into the body through the intestines. At this writing there are no standard dose guidelines for bromelain, however it is common for patients to take up to 320mg three times daily; this enzyme works best when taken on an empty stomach. *Precautions: Bromelain may decrease appetite. Do not use if you are already experiencing diarrhea. May cause rapid heartbeat and heavy menstrual periods. May affect patients who are allergic to carrots, celery, rye, wheat, latex, and bee venom. May interact with certain antibiotics, blood thinners, and some cancer agents, therefore do not use without consulting with your oncologist first.*

BU ZHONG YI QI*:*

This Chinese herbal formula also goes by the Korean name of Bojungikki-Tang and the Japanese name Hochueekkito. This formula contains the herbs astragalus root (*Astragalus membranaceus*), licorice root (*Glycyrrhiza glabra*), Asian ginseng (*Panax ginseng*), ginger root (*Zingiber officinale*), dong quai (*Angelica sinensis*),

---

163 Broccoli sprouts have 20-50 times more sulforaphane than fully mature broccoli heads.
164 *Properties and Therapeutic Application of Bromelain: A Review.* (Pavan, 2012)

citrus peels, red dates (*Ziziphus jujuba*), atractylodes (*Rhizoma atractylodis macrocephalae*), black cohosh (*cimicifuga racemosa*), and bupleurum (*Bupleurum falcatum*). This formula has been shown in clinical trials to significantly reduce cancer-related fatigue,[165] alleviate cachexia in animal studies,[166] accelerate recovery from leukopenia caused by cyclophosphamide,[167] and has been shown to be useful to use along with the chemotherapy agent gefitinib.[168] Because this is a complex formula I hesitate to provide general dose guidelines here; I strongly recommend that you seek the advice of a properly qualified practitioner of Traditional Chinese Medicine to receive dosage information. *Precautions: Because this formula has so many ingredients you must be sure to inquire whether any of them may work against your conventional treatment plan. Take note that some of the ingredients, such as dong quai, licorice, and black cohosh, may not be suitable for patients with an estrogen-fueled cancer. This formula may stimulate the immune system; seek your doctor's advice if you are on any therapy which either suppresses or stimulates the immune system.*

CAFFEINE:

Caffeine is a compound found naturally in dietary sources such as coffee, black tea, green tea, white tea, cocoa and chocolate. Herbal sources of caffeine include guarana (*Pallinia cupana*), yerba mate (*Ilex paraguariensis*), and kola nut (*Cola acuminata/C. nitida*). In 1991 the World Health Organization (WHO) announced that coffee consumption may increase the risk of developing bladder cancer and thus it was put on a list of possible carcinogens. Over time, however, scientific research has shown that not only was this incorrect, but coffee actually *helps reduce* the risk of various cancers and can help fight existing cancers. As a result, in 2016 WHO reversed their stance and announced "*[Scientists] found no conclusive evidence for a carcinogenic effect of drinking coffee.*"[169] [170] One study observed colon cancer patients[171] who drank at least 4 cups of coffee per day (460mg caffeine) were 42% less likely to experience the return of their cancer and 34% more likely to survive.[172] One study showed that the caffeine and caffeic acids in coffee significantly reduced the size of breast cancer tumors (both ER+ and ER-), lowered levels of IGF-1,[173] and

---

165 *Bojungikki-Tang For Cancer-Related Fatigue: A Pilot Randomized Clinical Trial.* (Jeong, 2010)

166 *Huchuekkito (TJ-41), a Kampo Formula, Ameliorates Cachexia Induced by Colon 26 Adenocarcinoma in Mice.* (Yae, 2012)

167 *Accelerated Recovery From Cyclophosphamide-induced Leukopenia in Mice Administered a Japanese Ethical Herbal Drug, Hochuekkito* (Kaneko, 1999)

168 *Effects of Bojungikki (A Polyherbal Formula) on Gefitinib Pharmacokinetics in Rats.* (Hyun, 2015)

169 *International Agency for Research on Cancer, World Health Organization, press release, June 15, 2016*

170 However, the study does go on to state that the drinking of very hot beverages in general may contribute to the risk of developing esophageal cancer, i.e. it is the temperature of the beverage that matters, not the drinks themselves.

171 These patients were also treated with surgery and/or chemotherapy.

172 Dana-***Farber Cancer Institute,*** news release, August 17, 2015: Drinking Coffee Daily May Improve Survival in Colon Cancer Patients.

173 IGF-1 a.ka. **I**nsulin-like **G**rowth **F**actor 1. This is a hormone produced in the pituitary gland

enhanced the activity of the chemotherapy agent tamoxifen. This effect was most pronounced on those who drank 4-5 cups per day.[174] Another study, using lung cancer cells, noted that caffeine enhanced the effects of the chemotherapeutic agent cisplatin in inducing cancer cell suicide.[175] Caffeine also has the ability to cross the blood-brain barrier making it a good candidate for adjuvant brain cancer therapy. One study observed that caffeine inhibits the movement of glioblastoma brain cancers thus reducing the risk of metastasis and increasing patient survival rates.[176] A large cohort study observed that people who drank caffeinated coffee or tea on a regular basis had a significantly lower rate of gliomas and meningiomas than patients who did not drink these caffeinated beverages.[177] If you are interested in using caffeine as a supportive treatment against your cancer be sure you use only natural sources of caffeine in your diet; avoid all artificial products such as soft drinks, energy shots, and the like. If you choose cocoa powder for your caffeine be aware that cocoa labeled "natural process" has significantly more healthful polyphenols than Dutch process cocoa. All caffeinated beverages should be consumed plain (no added sugars, dairy, flavorings, etc.) as the added creams and sugars will interfere with the benefits of the beverage. Here is a list of some natural products with the average amounts of caffeine they contain. Be aware that different brands may contain varying amounts. Consult with the individual commercial company to get an accurate milligram count on the product(s) you are using:

Coffee, brewed (8 oz.)	200mg caffeine
Coffee, instant (8 oz.)	173 mg caffeine
Black tea, brewed (8 oz.)	70 mg caffeine
Green tea (8 oz.)	45 mg caffeine
Iced tea (instant or bottled)	45 mg caffeine
White tea (8 oz.)	28 mg caffeine
Dark chocolate (1 oz.)	12 mg caffeine
Cocoa powder (1 oz.)	12 mg caffeine

Precautions: Do not consume caffeine six hours before bedtime to reduce your risk of insomnia. Do not consume more than 460mg of caffeine daily as too much may cause heart palpitations. Do not use caffeine if you have any type of heart arrhythmia issues. Overuse may cause anxiety, nervousness, and sweating. Natural dietary sources may contain antioxidants therefore consult with your oncologist to be sure the antioxidants will not interfere with your prescribed treatment regimen.

(located in the brain). In some individuals this hormone may raise the risk of certain cancers.

174 *Caffeine and Caffeic Acid Inhibit Growth and Modify Estrogen Receptor And Insulin-like Growth Factor 1 Receptor Levels in Human Breast Cancer.* (Rosendahl, 2015)

175 *The Effect of Caffeine on Cisplatin-induced Apoptosis of Lung Cancer Cells.* (Wang, 2015).

176 *Inhibition of the Ca^{2+} release channel, IP_3R subtype 3 by caffeine slows glioblastoma invasion and migration and extends survival.* (Kang, 2010)

177 *Coffee and Tea Intake and Risk of Brain Tumors in the European Prospective Investigation into Cancer and Nutrition Cohort Study.* (Michaud, 2010)

CALENDULA :

Calendula officinalis

Also known as pot marigold; do not confuse with other types of marigolds. Calendula is astringent, meaning it helps close open sores, but it also has mucilage which helps soothe inflamed tissues. These properties make it popular as a mouthwash or gargle when you have open sores in your mouth. Dosage: To make calendula tea use 2 tsp. (10ml) dried herb to 1 cup (240ml) of boiling water, steeped for 10 minutes and strained, or use 10 drops of tincture in ¼ cup (60ml)of water. Drink up to three times daily. This may also be used as a mouth rinse or a gargle. *Precautions: Do not use if you are allergic to plants in the ragweed family. May increase drowsiness caused by anesthesia or other surgical medications, so discontinue use at least two weeks before surgery. May also cause excessive drowsiness when used alongside other sedative medications or herbs.*

CANNABIS:

Cannabis sativa

This herb is commonly known as "marijuana" and is illegal to use in many areas, therefore you must check your local laws before using. If you live in an area where this herb is illegal you can still speak with your doctor about *legal* prescription medications which contain the same active ingredients contained in cannabis. Cannabis is well-known for increasing appetite, decreasing pain, and decreasing nausea.[178] The primary active substance is a cannabinoid known as THC,[179] a chemical which activates receptors in the brain that regulate pain, nausea and appetite; another cannabinoid in the herb, known as cannabidiol, ("CBD") regulates sensations of pain. Current research has also observed that both THC[180] and CBD[181] induce cell death in breast cancer cells, and CBD also inhibits tumor blood vessel formation.[182] Both of these cannabinoids have been observed to have synergistic effect with chemotherapy agents such as gemcitabine[183] and temozolomide,[184] creating a more effective outcome than with the chemotherapy medications alone. If such a tandem treatment is recommended for you then you should be aware that there is the risk of your cancer cells developing a resistance to the cannabinoids which may render the cannabis useless after a while. Although one of the more popular ways to consume this herb is to inhale its smoke you need to know the chemical changes caused by burning the herb creates substances which are very damaging to the lungs and can promote other cancers. One such substance is benzo-alpha-pyrene (BAP), a

---

178 *The Therapeutic Potential of Cannabis and Cannabinoids.* (Grotenhermen, 2012)

179 Also known as delta-9 tetrahydrocannabinol, also written as Δ^9- tetrahydrocannabinol.

180 *"Δ^9-Tetrahydrocannabinol Inhibits Cell Cycle Progression in Human Breast Cancer Cells through Cdc2 Regulation* (Caffarel, 2006)

181 *Cannabidiol Induces Programmed Cell Death in Breast Cancer Cells by Coordinating the Crosstalk between Apoptosis and Autophagy* (Shrivastava, 2011)

182 *Cannabidiol inhibits angiogenesis by multiple mechanisms* (Solinas, 2012)

183 *Gemcitabine/cannabinoid combination triggers autophagy in pancreatic cancer cells through a ROS-mediated mechanism.* (Donadelli, 2011)

184 *A combined preclinical therapy of cannabinoids and temozolomide against glioma.* (Torres, 2011)

chemical known for changing the tumor-suppression p53 gene, resulting in potential for cancer growth. What's worse, the THC acts synergistically with the BAP in the smoke, strengthening its ability to alter the p53 gene! Therefore, instead of smoking the herb it is much safer to consume it in edible form where it is legal, or use the purified cannabinoids in FDA-approved prescription medications. Take note that oral consumption of cannabis-based products may take up to an hour to feel the effects. In order to reduce the risk of over-consuming whole herb cannabis-based products you should buy only from reputable, legal, manufacturers who have standardized doses, and do not consume more than the amounts recommended by your oncologist or practitioner. Overdose symptoms include: disorientation, decreased coordination, dizziness, changes in heartbeat, panic attack, loss of contact with reality, and seizures. To prevent overdose here are some general guidelines (use only with competent professional guidance): **2.5mg** THC; encourages the appetite and may cause intoxication similar to a single serving of wine or beer; **5mg** THC; greatly increases the appetite and may cause intoxication similar to three servings of wine or beer; **10mg** THC; reduces pain and nausea., though this level results in significant intoxication. Because cannabinoids are fat soluble I strongly advise that you consume a little bit of heart-healthy fats along with your cannabis product (nuts, sunflower seeds, vegetable oil, etc.) in order for the cannabinoids to absorb properly in your system. If you are concerned about gauging your dosage, even if you are living in an area where cannabis is legal, you should discuss with your doctor about using cannabis-based prescription medications which are precisely measured. *Precautions: Do not over-consume any cannabis products as these pose the risk of intoxication. Many patients may develop resistance to the active substances. Due to the mind-altering effects of this herb do not consume any cannabis products if you expect to drive, operate heavy machinery, care for children or disabled/elderly adults, or otherwise need to maintain concentration or alertness. Keep all cannabis products out of reach of children and pets. Do not use if you have heart, lung, liver, or kidney disease. Do not use if you have a history of psychosis. May interact with other medications; check with your prescribing physicians.*

CAROB:
Catatonia siliqua

Carob is commonly used as a chocolate substitute for people with dietary sensitivities towards chocolate. It is derived from the podded seeds of the carob tree and is often sold in a form that looks like cocoa powder or chunky chocolate and is thus used in the same way as regular cocoa power or chunked chocolate. In some areas you may also see whole fresh or dried carob pods offered for sale; these pods are also edible. The tannins and mucilage in carob are well-known to have a significant calming effect on heartburn and diarrhea and may also help reduce vomiting. *Precautions: May lower blood sugar. As of this writing there are no known side effects or medication reactions associated with carob. People with nut or legume allergies may also be allergic to carob; be cautious.*

CAT'S CLAW:
Uncaria tomentosa

Cat's claw, a woody vine native to Central and South America, is named for its curved thorns located along its vines. Do not confuse it with the poisonous plant *acacia greggi,* which is also known as cat's claw, or the herb Devil's claw (*Harpagophytum procumbens*). Cat's claw is well-known for its ability to reduce inflammation and is also known for its ability to increase white blood cell counts, thus enhancing immune function. If you are on an immune-stimulating or immune-suppressing regimen consult with your prescribing physician before using cat's claw. Clinical trials have shown that water-based extracts of cat's claw enhance DNA repair of healthy cells after chemotherapy-induced DNA damage[185] and that breast cancer patients using the herb maintained better levels of infection-fighting white blood cells.[186] Cat's claw should by used only *after* a chemotherapy cycle is finished because taking it *during* the cycle risks repairing the DNA of the cancer cells along with your healthy cells. In vitro studies observed that cat's claw inhibits the growth of medullary thyroid cancer through cell death.[187] Another in vitro study observed that a compound known as mitraphylline in cat's claw, which can cross the blood-brain barrier, has significant action against neuroblastoma and glioma cells.[188] Other research has found that the quinovic acid glycosides and oxindole alkaloids from cat's claw has been shown to cause cell death in T24 an RT4 human bladder cancer cells.[189] [190] Intravesical administration (direct insertion into the bladder) may be advised. This herb is also known to improve the quality of life in patients with advanced solid tumors.[191] Studies have also shown that cat's claw inhibits production of **T**umor **N**ecrosis **F**actor, (TNF),[192] a cytokine which, when produced over a length of time, may contribute to cachexia.[193] This herb is best taken between meals. The following dosages are a general guideline: *Tincture*: Take according to package directions with ½ cup (120ml) of water and a tablespoon (15ml) of lemon juice, as it needs the acid from the juice to help release the effective agents. *Root bark extract:* Take up to 350mg of the extract daily. Extract should be standardized to at least 8% carboxy alkyl esters and less than 0.5% oxindole alkaloids. Take with ½ cup (120ml) of water

---

185 *DNA Repair Enhancement of water-based Extracts of Uncaria Tomentosa in a Human Volunteer Study* (Y. Sheng, 2001)

186 *Uncaria tomentosa-Adjuvant Treatment for Breast Cancer: Clinical Trial.* (Santos Araújo , 2010)

187 *Antiproliferative and pro-apoptotic effects of Uncaria tomentosa in human medullary thyroid carcinoma cells.* (Rinner, 2009)

188 *Antiproliferative effects of mitraphylline, a pentacyclic oxindole alkaloid of Uncaria tomentosa on human glioma and neuroblastoma cell lines.* (Prado, 2007)

189 *Quinovic Acid Glycosides Purified Fraction from Uncaria Tomentosa Induces Cell Death by Apoptosis in the T24 Human Bladder Cancer Cell Line* (Dietrich, 2014)

190 *Cat's claw oxindole alkaloid isomerization induced by cell incubation and cytotoxic activity against T24 and RT4 human bladder cancer cell lines.* (Kaiser, 2013)

191 *Uncaria tomentosa (cat's claw) improves quality of life in patients with advanced solid tumors.* (de Paula, 2015)

192 *Cat's claw inhibits TNFα production and scavenges free radicals: role in cytoprotection* (Manuel Sandoval, 2000)

193 *Tumor necrosis factor-α and Muscle Wasting: A Cellular Perspective*(Michael B. Reid, 2001)

and a tablespoon (15ml) of lemon juice, as it needs the acid from the lemon juice to help release the effective agents. *Whole root bark:* Make a decoction by simmering 4-5 pieces of the bark in one quart of water (960ml) for fifteen minutes. Strain out the bark and cool the decoction. Add one tablespoon of lemon juice. Drink one cup, (240ml) up to three time daily. *Capsules:* These should have the pentacylic form of this herb, with a minimum of 1.3% pentacylic oxindole alkaloids and no tetracylic oxindole alkaloids. Use according to package directions. *Precautions: Do not use cat's claw if you are diabetic. May cause dizziness, nausea, and diarrhea. May interfere with controlling blood pressure after surgery, therefore discontinue use for two weeks before surgery May cause stomach and bowel discomfort. May lower blood pressure. May cause kidney failure in patients with systemic lupus erythematosus. May worsen the symptoms of Parkinson's disease. May increase the effect of blood thinners Increases blood levels of atazanavir, ritonavir, and saquinavir medications. May stimulate the immune system therefore you must avoid use if you've had an organ or bone marrow transplant or suffer from an autoimmune disease. Side effects include dizziness, headaches, and vomiting. Do not use if you have leukemia. May interact with medications that are processed by the liver.*

CLARY SAGE:
Salvia sclarea

Do not confuse with sage leaf (*Salvia officinalis*). Some patients avoid clary sage oil because they are told it is estrogenic due to the presence of a substance called sclareol, which is structurally similar to human estrogens. However, in vitro research has shown that it is effective against breast and uterine cancers with action similar to the chemotherapy agent tamoxifen.[194] Aside from this issue, other in vitro research has also shown sclareol to be effective against some human leukemia cell lines[195] and osteosarcoma lines,[196] however clinical studies have not yet been established as of this writing. Aside from these concerns, clary sage oil has also been shown to be highly effective in killing several strains of antibiotic-resistant staph infections on the skin.[197] Clary sage also contains substances which reduce depression[198] feelings of stress and anxiety. It is also a mild sedative to help promote sleep. One clinical trial observed that clary sage oil may be more useful than lavender oil in reducing blood pressure.[199] One popular recipe for a relaxing bath blend: 3 drops of clary sage with 2 drops of ylang ylang. *Precautions: Some practitioners may recommend applying the oil on the*

194 *Cell growth inhibitory action of an unusual labdane diterpene, 13-epi-sclareol in breast and uterine cancers in vitro.* (Sashidhara, 2007)
195 *The effect of sclareol on growth and cell cycle progression of human leukemic cell lines.* (Dimas, 2006)
196 *Sclareol, a plant diterpene, exhibits potent antiproliferative effects via the induction of apoptosis and mitochondrial membrane potential loss in osteosarcoma cancer cells.* (Wang, 2015)
197 *The effect of clary sage oil on staphylococci responsible for wound infections.* (Sienkiewicz, 2015)
198 *Changes in 5-hydroxytryptamine and cortisol plasma levels in menopausal women after inhalation of clary sage oil.* (Lee, 2014)
199 *Randomized Controlled Trial for Salvia sclarea or Lavandula angustifolia: Differential Effects on Blood Pressure in Female Patients with Urinary Incontinence Undergoing Urodynamic Examination* (Seol, 2013)

skin undiluted ("neat"). However, applying essential oils neat may cause sensitivity; use neat with caution. To use it diluted, place 12 drops of clary sage oil in 30ml (2 tablespoons) of vegetable oil or mineral oil. Do not use internally without competent professional guidance.

CHLOROPHYLL:

Chlorophyll is a natural green pigment found in all green plants. Many people believe that chlorophyll, which has an atomic structure closely matching hemoglobin in red blood cells,[200] can help build up the number of red blood cells in a person's system. Although chlorophyll and hemoglobin molecules *are* very similarly structured they are not interchangeable: The primary difference is the presence of iron in hemoglobin, which is necessary for the blood cells to be able to transport oxygen. Since chlorophyll does *not* contain any iron it cannot carry oxygen to your body's cells as hemoglobin would. Therefore, chlorophyll is not a good option for boosting red blood cell counts. As for chlorophyll's known ability to fight cancer, take note that Oregon State University published a study on rainbow trout that found chlorophyll can be protective against modest levels of cancer-causing agents, however, when pitted against very high levels of cancer-causing agents chlorophyll actually *increased* the number of tumors formed.[201] It is unknown at this time how this may translate to human cancer activity.

CLOVES:

Eugenia Caryophyllata / Syzygium aromaticum

Do not confuse with garlic cloves (*Allium sativum*). Studies have shown that eugenol, a substance in cloves, can inhibit the production of interleukins, a family of cytokines known to contribute to inflammation and cachexia[202] and other studies have shown eugenol to induce cancer cell death and inhibit tumor blood vessel formation.[203] Cloves are also useful in reducing the incidence of nausea and vomiting.

Some studies have also shown eugenol to be effective in inhibiting the growth of melanoma and therefore some holistic practitioners recommend applying clove oil to skin cancer lesions. *However,* two things must be taken into consideration: Number one, pure clove oil is highly toxic and must be diluted in a carrier oil before being applied to the skin (12 drops of clove oil in 30ml [2 tablespoons] of vegetable oil or mineral oil). Number two, do not use clove oil on skin cancers without discussing it with your oncologist or other holistic practitioners first. This is because the oil may interfere with some topical prescription medications or may interfere with other holistic methods that are applied to the skin. To use whole cloves drink 1 cup (240ml)

---

200 Both have a ring structure with nearly the exact same ions. Hemoglobin has an iron ion in the center, chlorophyll has a magnesium ion in the center.

201 News release: *"Chlorophyll Can Help Prevent Cancer – But Study Raises Other Questions"* Oregon State University, January 12, 2012

202 *Clove and eugenol in noncytotoxic concentrations exert immunomodulatory/anti-inflammatory action on cytokine production by murine macrophages* (Bachiega, 2012)

203 *Eugenol Induces Apoptosis and Inhibits Invasion and Angiogenesis in a Rat Model of Gastric Carcinogenesis Induced by MNNG.* (Manikandan, 2010)

of clove tea three times daily. Recipe: Bring 4 cups (960ml) of hot water to a boil, then turn down the heat to a low simmer. Put 9 whole cloves or ¾ tsp (4ml) ground cloves into the hot water. Let simmer for 5 minutes. Strain and drink. *Precautions: Use only whole cloves or ground cloves, do not substitute for clove oil; clove oil is highly concentrated and quickly becomes toxic when used internally. Cloves thin the blood* .

COENZYME Q10:

Also known as CoQ10, this is a natural substance produced by your body to create the energy needed for cell growth. One study was published which suggested that CoQ10 administered during treatment with anthracyclines such as doxorubicin and daunorubicin reduces the risk of heart damage[204] and another study observed it helped protect the testicles from damage caused by doxorubicin in mouse models.[205] In a series of case studies of five different breast cancer patients it was observed that patients given 390mg of CoQ10 daily during conventional treatment experienced significant regression of tumors and reversal of metastasis.[206] *Precautions: CoQ10 is an antioxidant and may not be suitable for your particular treatment regimen. Speak with your doctor about this treatment before taking any supplements. Some patients experience nausea, diarrhea, and loss of appetite with this supplement. Do not use CoQ10 supplements if you are on blood thinners or theophylline due to the potential for dangerous interaction.*

COFFEE ENEMAS:
See also "Caffeine" in this chapter

Coffee enemas became popular in the 1930's when Dr. Max Gerson began using them as an alternative treatment for his cancer patients. According to Gerson, coffee enemas work by activating antioxidant enzymes which detoxify waste products from the cancer tumor's cells. It is also taught by many practitioners that the caffeine in the coffee dilates the patient's bile ducts promoting clearance of toxins from the liver, stimulates removal of toxins in the blood into the bowel, and stimulates the digestive system to clear any toxins from the gut; however, there is no scientific evidence showing that coffee can affect liver and gall bladder activity. Coffee is known to be rich in antioxidants, and clinical studies have suggested that *drinking* coffee in moderation (2-4 cups per day) may reduce consumers' risk of developing colorectal cancer, liver cancer, and uterine cancer. Newer research has shown that coffee is also beneficial in reducing inflammation in the body. This is certainly good news for coffee drinkers, but what about the idea of using coffee as an *enema* to treat cancer? Clinical studies have been performed to investigate this very question. One

---

204 *Coenzyme Q10 for Prevention of Anthracycline-Induced Cardiotoxicity* (Conklin, 2005).

205 *Protective mechanisms of coenzyme-Q10 may involve up-regulation of testicular P-glycoprotein in doxorubicin-induced toxicity.* (El-Sheikh, 2014) Dosage was 15mg of CoQ10 per kg of body weight, once daily, orally, starting on the fourth day of doxorubicin treatment, ongoing for eight days.

206 *Progress on therapy of breast cancer with vitamin Q10 and the regression of metastases.* (Lockwood, 1995)

study compared the antioxidant effects of an orally administered cup of coffee versus a coffee enema and found there was no difference in blood levels of antioxidant activity.[207] Another study compared the absorption of caffeine in a cup of coffee versus absorption from a coffee enema and found that *oral* consumption of coffee resulted in a *significantly higher absorption* of caffeine than from an enema.[208] Clearly the digestion of coffee in the stomach does not hinder the absorption of antioxidants and caffeine. It also should also be noted that the acidic properties of coffee are better handled in the stomach than in the colon and rectum. Since oral consumption of coffee allows the same amount of antioxidant absorption and better absorption of caffeine than the enema method, this make the enema method completely unnecessary. And, not only is the enema method unnecessary, it is also known to be unsafe. Coffee enemas are well-known to risk causing bowel punctures and burns in the bowel lining allowing opportunity for a serious infection to take hold. I strongly advise you to decline coffee enema treatments and simply treat yourself to a a few cups of (black) coffee instead.

CONJUGATED LINOLEIC ACID:

Conjugated Linoleic Acid, (CLA) is mixture of different forms of linoleic acid, an essential fatty acid. Sources of CLA include beef, lamb, diary, and crimini mushrooms; it can also be purchased as a dietary supplement. In vitro studies have shown CLA to inhibit estrogenic activity in ER+ breast cancer cells,[209] inhibit tumor blood vessel formation in ER+ breast cancer cells,[210] and may reduce the spread and treatment resistance of rectal cancers in patients undergoing chemo-radiotherapy.[211] The typical recommended dose of CLA is 3-5 g daily. *Precautions: Patients with cardiovascular issues or diabetes should use caution when using products containing CLA. Side effects from CLA use include fatigue and digestive issues and may thin the blood. Use of CLA may increase the risk of developing diabetes if you have metabolic syndrome.*

COPTIS:

Coptis chinensis

This herb is also known in TCM as Huanglian or goldenthread; do not confuse this with other herbs known by similar names such as three-leaf goldenthread (*Coptis trifolia*), golden root (*Scutellaria baikalensis* or *Rhodiola Rosea*), or goldenseal (*Hydrastis*

---

207 *Antioxidant Effects After Coffee Enema or Coffee Consumption in Healthy Thai Male Volunteers* (Teekachunhatean, 2012)

208 *Pharmacokinetics of Caffeine following a Single Administration of Coffee Enema versus Oral Coffee Consumption in Healthy Male Subjects* (Teekachunhatean, 2013)

209 *Conjugated Linoleic Acid Blocks Estrogen Signaling in Human Breast Cancer Cells.* (Tanmahasamut,, 2004)

210 *Anti-angiogenesis Effects of Conjugated Linoleic Acid in Human Breast Cancer Cell Line MCF-7* (Li-Shu Wang, 2004)

211 *Effect of conjugated linoleic acid supplementation on inflammatory factors and matrix metalloproteinase enzymes in rectal cancer patients undergoing chemoradiotherapy.,* (Mohammedzadeh, 2013)

canadensis).[212] Since coptis contains berberine please also see "berberine" in this chapter. In vitro studies have shown coptis to enhance the effects of agents used for treating ER+ breast cancers (specifically tamoxifen and fulvestrant).[213] According to certified nutritional consultant and author Phyllis A. Balch, applying a cold compress of coptis to one's skin 2-3 times daily will help increase the absorption of topical 5-FU for skin cancer.[214] *Whole herb:* Make a decoction with a ratio of 1 teaspoon (15ml) of whole herb per 1 cup (240ml) of water. Before adding the herb bring the water to a boil, then add the herb. Turn the water down to a simmer and let heat for 15 minutes. Turn off the heat, strain out the herb, and let the decoction cool. Drink one cup of decoction up to four times daily. *Tincture:* Place 30 drops of tincture into ½ cup (120ml) of water; drink up to four times per day. *Extract:* Take according to package directions. *Capsules:* Take according to package directions. *Precautions: Do not use coptis if you are jaundiced. May lower blood pressure. Do not exceed recommended dosage. Do not take for prolonged periods of time. May cause jaundice in children or those with liver problems. Do not use if you have heart disease. May cause nausea.*

DANDELION:
Taraxacum officinale

Dandelion root is well-known for being a protective liver tonic and is often recommended for protection against the toxic effects of chemotherapy agents on the liver. Although studies which specifically focus on dandelion's protection against chemotherapy-induced liver damage are lacking, numerous other studies do show dandelion root to be protective of the liver in many other cases of chemically induced damages such as alcohol and carbon tetrachloride.[215] [216] Therefore I highly recommend that you speak to your doctor regarding this herb if you are looking to protect your liver. If you choose to use this herb, typical dosing is as follows: Boil 2 teaspoons (10ml) of dried dandelion root in 1 ½ cups (180ml) water for 10 minutes. Strain and drink up to three times daily. *Precautions: Patients with bile duct obstruction must use caution. May have mild side effects such as indigestion or low blood sugar. Use caution if you are allergic to plants in the ragweed family. May interact with certain antibiotics, lithium, diuretics, or medications changed by the liver. Do not use if you have had an organ transplant or kidney disease. Ethanol*

---

212 *C. chinensis, C. trifolia,* and *H. canadensis* are related plants however, there are differences: *H. canadensis* contains the most berberine, *C. trifolia* contains the most coptisine, and *H. canadensis* & *C. chinensis* uniquely contain hydrastine and palmatine among the three species. Due to the differences in these constituents these plants are not always interchangeable in use. [*Significant Differences in Alkaloid Content of Coptis chinensis (Huanglian), From its Related American Species.* (Kamath, 2009)]

213 *Coptis extracts enhance the anticancer effect of estrogen receptor antagonists on human breast cancer cells* (Liu Jing, 2009)

214 Book: ***Prescription for Herbal Healing***, p.222, Phyllis A. Balch, 2012

215 *In vitro and in vivo hepatoprotective effects of the water-based extract from Taraxacum officinale (dandelion) root against alcohol-induced oxidative stress* (You, 2010)

216 *Hepatoprotective Effect of Dandelion (Taraxacum Officinale) Against Induced Chronic Liver Cirrhosis* (Al-Malki, 2013)

extracts of dandelion may have estrogenic effect, therefore look for non-alcohol extracts. May have diuretic effect.

DEVIL'S CLAW:

Harpagophytum procumbens

Not to be confused with the herb Cat's claw (*Uncaria tomentosa*), or the poisonous plant *acacia greggi* which is also known as devil's claw and/or cat's claw. *H. procumbens* is a relative of the sesame seed plant (*Sesamum indicum*); although I have found no evidence that this plant can trigger a response in patients allergic to sesame products one needs to assess the risk for oneself. This herb is named for the claw-like appearance of its fruit, though it is the root parts which are used therapeutically. Devil's claw contains harpagoside, a substance which reduces inflammation. In vivo studies show that devil's claw can inhibit the production of interleukins[217] and TNF,[218] cytokines known to contribute to cachexia. This can be beneficial for patients who are experience inflammation-induced pain or cachexia during their treatments. Because of this effect on the immune system I strongly advise you to speak with your prescribing physicians first if you are on any kind of therapy which either stimulates or suppresses the immune system. Beyond its anti-inflammatory properties two case studies side by side strongly suggested the use of devil's claw in the regression of follicular lymphoma.[219] Typical dosage: Up to 1,200 mg daily in divided doses. Make sure your commercial preparations are standardized to contain 2-3% iridoid glycosides. Taken as an extract, effective dosing of devil's claw means taking 50-100 mg harpagoside daily, divided into three doses, for 2-4 months. Taken as a tea: Pour 12 oz. (360 ml) of boiling water over 1 teaspoon (5ml) of devil's claw root and steep for eight hours. Divide into three portions and drink throughout the day. *Precautions: Contains antioxidants, so be sure you are not undergoing a therapy that requires avoidance of high antioxidants. Use may increase risk of developing pancreatitis. May cause stomach issues in some patients. Has blood thinning properties. May lower blood sugar. May decrease the effectiveness of antacids due to increased production of stomach acids. May cause blood pressure changes. Safety of long term use is unknown. May increase bile production, do not use if you have gall bladder problems.*

ECHINACEA:

Echinacea purpurea/ Echinacea angustifolia/ Echinacea pallida

Echinacea, also known as purple coneflower, is commonly used for boosting the immune system for a variety of illnesses. Although echinacea is purported to be a strong immunity booster evidence is mixed as to whether this is true. This is primarily

---

217*Inhibitory effects of devil's claw (secondary root of Harpagophyperthermia therapyum procumbens) extract and harpagoside on cytokine production in mouse macrophages* (K. Inaba, 2010)

218*Molecular Targets of the Anti inflammatory Harpagophyperthermia therapyum Procumbens (Devil's Claw): Inhibition of TNFα and COX-2 Gene Expression by Preventing Activation of AP-1* (Bernd L. Fiebich, 2012)

219 *Regression of follicular lymphoma with Devil's Claw: coincidence or causation?* (Wilson, 2009)

due to the fact the various studies do not use a singular "version" of echinacea. Medical echinacea comes in two species, and different parts of the plant of each species (flowers, leaves, and roots) contain varying amounts of healing agents. Along with that there are the various ways the herb is prepared: As a tea, a tincture, a capsule, a tablet, etc. Each of these factors influence the outcome of a clinical trial, and this is why there are conflicting reports. The aerial parts of the plant (leaves and stems) tend to contain the highest levels of the immune-boosting substances. In Germany, where the government regulates herbal medicines, echinacea's aerial parts are approved for treating upper respiratory infections, urinary tract infections, and wounds. Be aware that, if you are on any kind of immune-modulating therapies you should discuss this herb with your prescribing physicians before using echinacea for internal illnesses. For topical fungal infections echinacea has been shown to be useful in clearing them up. Since some cancer patients find themselves more susceptible to contracting fungal infections due to reduced immune system this can be good. Clinical trials have found that volunteers with yeast infections who combined echinacea juice with the anti-fungal cream econazole experienced only a 15% recurrence rate, compared to those using only econazole who experienced a 60% recurrence rate.[220] *Precautions: Do not use if you are allergic to plants in the ragweed family. Do not use if you have an autoimmune disorder. Echinacea may increase how long caffeine stays in your system before your body breaks it down. Do not use echinacea if you are taking any medications or chemotherapy agents which put your liver at risk.*

EMODIN:

This is a plant-based compound often found in rhubarb (*Rheum rhabarbarum*), buckthorn, (*Rhamnus cathartica*) aloe, (*Aloe vera*), and Japanese knotweed (*Fallopia japonica*) but it can also be taken as a prescription medication. It is used for reducing inflammation, as a potent laxative, and as a treatment for diabetes but is also used for reversing chemo-resistance in several types of cancers.[221] In vitro and in vivo studies have also observed emodin to inhibit the growth and metastases of many cancers,[222] and some studies have observed that combining emodin with curcumin, a pigment in the spice turmeric, causes a synergistic effect against breast cancer cells,[223] and cervical cancer.[224] Emodin has also been observed to enhance the action of

---

220 *Recurrent candidiasis: Adjuvant immunotherapy with different formulations of Echinacin®* (Coeugniet, 1986)

221 Some examples: *Emodin enhances cytotoxicity of chemotherapeutic drugs in prostate cancer cells: The mechanisms involve ROS-mediated suppression of multi-drug resistance and hypoxia inducible factor-1* (Huang, 2008); *Emodin reverses gemcitabine resistance in pancreatic cancer cells via the mitochondrial apoptosis pathway in vitro* (Liu, 2012); *Emodin sensitizes paclitaxel-resistant human ovarian cancer cells to paclitaxel-induced apoptosis in vitro.*(Li, 2009)

222 *Anthraquinone emodin inhibits human cancer cell invasiveness by antagonizing P2X7 receptors* (Jelassi, 2013); Book: **Sensitization of Cancer Cells for Chemo/Immuno/Radio-therapy**, pp. 222-223, Edited by Benjamin Bonavida, PhD

223 *Synergistic effects of curcumin with emodin against the proliferation and invasion of breast cancer cells through upregulation of miR-34a.* (Guo, 2013);

224 *Curcumin and Emodin Down-Regulate TGF-β Signaling Pathway in Human Cervical Cancer*

chemotherapy agents such as cisplatin,[225] and, when combined with DHA, has been observed to enhance the chemotherapy combination treatment of arsenic trioxide and interferon- α against leukemia.[226] *Precautions: Over-use of this substance may cause severe diarrhea, nausea, and vomiting; use only with competent supervision. Use only for short periods of time. May decrease the effectiveness of aspirin therapy for heart patients. Do not use alcohol during emodin treatment. Do not use for two weeks before or two weeks after surgery. May interact with other medications; check with your prescribing physicians before use.*

ENGLISH LAVENDER:
Lavandula angustifolia / Lavandula officinalis

English lavender contains linalool and other substances shown in studies to effect the central nervous system in ways that calm and soothe.[227] therefore it is often used to help counteract anxiety and promote better sleep. Patients can either use the whole herb as a tea or use the essential oils as an aromatherapeutic agent. Use only English lavender as other forms of lavender may not work as well. English lavender has been shown to be effective in helping reduce anxiety in patients.[228] A study published in 2012 involving twenty participants showed that inhaling the scent from lavender oil, normally used for calming the mood, also decreased the participants' blood pressures and heart rates.[229] Do not use the oil on your skin undiluted ("neat") to reduce risk of developing skin sensitivity. Dilute 12 drops of oil in 2 tablespoons (30ml) of a carrier oil such as mineral oil or vegetable oil, or alternatively put 12 drops of oil into your plain bath water. You may also place 2 drops of oil in 2 cups of hot steamy water to use as steam inhalation therapy. To drink the herbal tea use 2 teaspoons (10ml) of whole herb steeped in 1 cup of boiling water. Strain and drink up to three times daily. To use the tincture: Take 20-40 drops of lavender tincture in ½ cup (120ml) of water up to three times daily. *Precautions: Do not use if you are allergic to any plants in the lavender family. May increase sedative effects of other medications when consumed orally. Do not use for two weeks before surgical procedures. Topical application may increase sun sensitivity. Excessive oral intake may cause nausea and vomiting.*

Cells (Thacker, 2015)

225 *Synergistic cancer growth-inhibitory effect of emodin and low-dose cisplatin on gastric cancer cells In vitro* (Huang, 2015)

226 *Emodin and DHA potently increase arsenic trioxide interferon-α–induced cell death of HTLV-I–transformed cells by generation of reactive oxygen species and inhibition of Akt and AP-1* (Brown, 2007)

227 *Lavender and the Nervous System.* (Koulivand, 2013) [Use only true lavender/English lavender, *Lavandula angustifolium.*]

228 *Lavender and the Nervous System.* (Koulivand, 2013) [Use only true lavender/English lavender, *Lavandula angustifolium.*]

229 ***Journal of the Medical Association of Thailand,*** April 2012, Vol. 95, No.4, pp.598-606 "*The Effects of Lavender Oil Inhalation On Emotional States, Autonomic Nervous System, and Brain Electrical Activity*", Winai Sayorwan

EPA :

Eicosapentaenoic acid

EPA is an Omega 3 fatty acid found in fish oils. A review of studies noted that use of EPA helped reduce the severity of cancer-related cachexia by reducing systemic inflammation.[230] In one small study involving 26 pancreatic cancer patients with cachexia it was observed that weight loss was stabilized and some even gained back some of their weight.[231] These studies should not be taken to mean that EPA cures cachexia, it simply means that it can help reduce the severity of the condition. Typical dosage of EPA fish oil supplements range from 3,000 - 4,000mg per day. There are no vegan sources of this supplement. *Precautions: Fish oil is a known blood thinner. May cause digestive upset. May lower blood sugar and blood pressure levels. Do not use if you are sensitive to salicylates such as aspirin, black haw (Viburnum prunifolium), cramp bark (Viburnum opulus), marshmallow root (althaea officinalis), meadowsweet (Filipendula ulmaria),* sweet birch *(Betula lenta),* white birch *(Betula papyrifera),* white *willow bark (salix alba), and wintergreen (Gaultheria procumbens). This is not a comprehensive list, consult with an experienced herbalist.*

EVODIA:

Evodia rutaecarpa

Evodia is a tree native to eastern Asia; its fruit is used in Traditional Chinese Medicine under the name "wuzhuyu." In studies on breast cancer cells a substance found in evodia, known as evodiamine, has been shown to reverse resistance to doxorubicin in animal models.[232] Other studies have also shown evodia to reduce metastasis and tumor blood vessel formation on several cancer cell lines in animal studies.[233] The best methods of absorption are using whole fruit or using ethanol extract. Taking evodia with coptis will increase the absorption of evodia however it will also decrease the absorption of the coptis. To make evodia tea: Bring 10 cups (2,400ml) of water to a boil in a pot. Add 1 ounce (28g) of evodia berries and immediately turn the water down to as low as possible, cover the pot, and keep heated on low for 20 minutes. Turn off the heat, strain out the berries and let the liquid cool. Divide the liquid into nine doses and refrigerate. Take three doses per day. If instead you use a commercial supplement then use according to package directions. *Precautions:This herb is known to interact with blood thinners, reduce the effects of caffeine and theophylline, and interacts with medications changed by the liver.*

FLAX SEED:

Linum usitatissimum

Flax seed, also known as linseed, is known for its mucilaginous properties and

---

230 *Eicosapentaenoic Acid in Cancer Improves Body Composition and Modulates Metabolism* (Pappalardo, 2015)

231 *Effect of Oral Eicosapentaenoic Acid on Weight Loss in Patients with Pancreatic Cancer* (Wigmore, 2000)

232 *Evodiamine Synergizes with Doxorubicin in the Treatment of Chemoresistant Human Breast Cancer without Inhibiting P-Glycoprotein* (Wang, 2014)

233 *Evodiamine: A Novel Anti-Cancer Alkaloid from Evodia rutaecarpa* (Jiang, 2009)

the ability to move stool through the bowel. It is also well-known for its abundance of omega 3 fatty acids, an important nutrient for heart health (see subheading "Omega 3 Fatty Acids" in this chapter). Whole flax seeds will pass through your digestive tract without changing, therefore you should buy it already ground or run the whole seeds through a grinder in order to derive benefit from the fatty acids. Because of its mucilage ground flax seed will thicken soups and other liquids it is added to. You may also want to mix it into your yogurt, sprinkle it on your hot cereal, or add a a couple of teaspoons into your favorite muffin recipe. *Precautions: Omega 3 fatty acids thin the blood, therefore it is advisable to use this product in moderation to prevent bleeding issues. Do not use if you are already taking blood thinners. Do not use the whole seed if you have diverticulitis or any inflammatory bowel disease.*

GARLIC:
Allium sativum

Raw garlic contains the substances alliinase and alliin which, when you crush garlic, mix together to create a therapeutic compound known as allicin. It takes about ten minutes after crushing the garlic for the allicin to completely form. In vitro studies have shown allicin to be an exceptionally effective agent against various kinds of cancer cells, however, allicin is very quickly metabolized in the human body and as yet there are no published studies showing whether it can remain in the human body long enough to affect cancer cells the same way. In spite of this, garlic has been shown in human trials to be helpful against cancer in other ways. For example, in one trial involving 50 patients with advanced cancers, those who were supplemented with aged garlic extract experienced increased natural killer cells activity.[234] One trial involving 51 patients showed that aged garlic extract suppresses the progression of colorectal adenomas (precancerous polyps in the bowel) in diagnosed patients.[235] Another trial involving 21 patients with basal cell carcinoma (a type of skin cancer) showed that topical application of ajoene, another constituent in garlic, caused cancer cell death resulting in reduced tumor size in 17 patients (80% of the participants).[236] Raw garlic is also a known anti-fungal agent. To treat fungal infections on the skin you should apply slices of raw garlic on the lesions for 6 hour intervals (with 6 hours rest in between intervals). The infection should clear up within 48 hours. Take note that the application of the raw garlic on the fungus lesions may cause temporary, minor discomfort in some patients. *Precautions: Garlic is a blood thinner.. May lower blood sugar and may reduce the effectiveness of some medications. Consuming raw garlic may cause stomach upset in sensitive people. Do not use if you are allergic to plants in the onion family. Raw garlic applied to the skin may cause blistering in some patients. Do not consume alcohol if you are taking garlic orally. May decrease the effectiveness of hormone-based birth control methods.*

234*Aged Garlic Extract Prevents a Decline of NK Cell Number and Activity in Patients With Advanced Cancer* (Ishikawa, 2006)

235 *Aged Garlic Extract Has Potential Suppressive Effect on Colorectal Adenomas in Humans* (Tanaka, 2006)

236*The garlic-derived organosulfur component ajoene decreases basal cell carcinoma tumor size by inducing apoptosis* (Tilli, 2003)

GERMAN CHAMOMILE:
Matricaria chamomilla[237]

Do not confuse with Roman chamomile (*Anthemis nobilis/Chamaemelum nobile*). German chamomile is commonly known to reduce anxiety and and promote sleep. This sedation is due to the presence of apigenin, a substance in the plant which binds to the same receptors in the brain affected by prescription sedatives such as Valium[238] (see also the subheading "apigenin" in this chapter). German chamomile is also known for its ability to heal skin problems and reduce inflammation. Since inflammation is usually due to an immune response I strongly advise you to check with your oncologist and other prescribing physicians first if you are on any kind of immune-suppression or immune-stimulation treatments. Anecdotal evidence shows that cancer patients experiencing mouth sores from certain chemotherapy agents have had success in reducing the discomfort and severity of mouth sores when using a chamomile tea gargle three times daily. Some patients experiencing insomnia find that drinking chamomile tea about an hour before bed helps alleviate the sleeplessness (though it can take up to four weeks of nightly tea to achieve full effect in some people). In vivo studies have shown that a tandem treatment with German chamomile and black cumin significantly protects the kidneys from the chemotoxic effects of cisplatin.[239] Research using mouse models observed that treated mice showed that German chamomile extract gave significant reduction in cisplatin-caused peripheral neuropathic pain and inflammation better than morphine.[240] German chamomile contains a substance called bisabololoxide-A. In vitro studies have shown that combining it with the chemotherapy agent 5-FU worked better against chronic myelogenous leukemia (CML) cells than 5-FU alone.[241] When using chamomile as an aromatherapy agent take note: Although German chamomile and Roman chamomile both give sedative and anti-inflammatory effects, their levels of healing agents are not matched. Therefore, Roman chamomile essential oils used in aromatherapy is a better calming agent and German chamomile oil is better as a topical agent against inflammation. Dosage: To drink as a tea steep 1 tablespoon (15ml) of dried flowerheads in 1 cup (240ml) of boiling water. Steep for 10 minutes, strain and drink. To use the oil as a topical agent mix 12 drops of German chamomile essential oil with 30ml (2 tablespoons) of carrier oil such as mineral oil or vegetable oil. *Precautions: Do not use Chamomile if you are allergic to plants in the ragweed family. Chamomile may interact with hormonal drugs, birth control pills, blood thinners, and sedative drugs. May interact with drugs processed by the liver. May increase blood levels of cyclosporine medications. May worsen asthma symptoms in some people.*

---

237 Synonyms include: *Matricaria recutita, Chamomilla chamomilla, Chamomilla recutita*, and *Matricaria suaveolens*.

238 Chamomile: A herbal medicine of the past with bright future. (Srivastava, 2010)

239 *Nephroprotective Effect of Nigella Sativa and Matricaria Chamomilla in Cisplatin Induced Renal Injury* (Ragaa Hamdy Mohamed Salama, 2011)

240 *Effect of Matricaria chamomilla Hydroalcoholic Extract on Cisplatin-induced Neuropathy in Mice.* (Abad, 2011)

241 *Cytoxic Action of Bisabololoxide-A of German Chamomile on Human Leukemia K562 Cells In Combination With 5-Fluorouracil.* (Ogata-Ikeda, 2011)

84

GINGER
Zingiber Officinale

Research using ginger on animal models has shown ginger to provide significant protection for the kidneys during chemotherapy treatments using the drugs cisplatin[242] and doxorubicin.[243] In numerous human studies ginger has been shown to be highly effective in reducing chemotherapy-induced nausea and systemic inflammation.[244] In vitro studies have shown ginger to reduce the viability of gastric cancer cells,[245] induce cell death in colorectal cancer cells,[246] and inhibits the growth of prostate cancer cells.[247] Other studies, both in vitro and in vivo show substances in ginger known as 6-Gingerol and zerumbone inhibit tumor blood vessel formation through inhibition of VEGF[248 249] as well as inhibiting the production of cytokines that are known to contribute to cachexia.[250] *Dosages*: Take a single dose up to three times daily. Because ginger comes in several forms here is a list of what a "single dose" is:

- 1 cup (240ml) of ginger tea
- 1 medium piece of crystallized ginger (1 inch square or 2.5 cm square)
- 2 droppers full of ginger extract
- 2 teaspoons of ginger syrup
- 1 tablespoon (15ml) freshly grated root
- ½ teaspoon (3ml) of ground ginger.

Precautions: Ginger is a blood thinner. Overuse may cause uterine contractions. Ginger can prolong the effect of barbituates. Do not use if you have gallstones, inflammatory bowel disease, irritable bowel syndrome, or ulcers. May lower blood sugar levels. May lower blood pressure. May worsen some heart conditions, especially arrhythmias – speak with your cardiologist.

GINKGO:
Ginkgo biloba

Studies have shown ginkgo to contain three flavonoids (kaempferol, quercetin, and isorhamnetin) which, when used together, inhibit estrogen production.[251] Since

242 *Zingiber officinale Roscoe alone and in combination with α-tocopherol protect the kidney against cisplatin-induced acute renal failure* (Ajith, 2007)

243 *Protective effect of Zingiber officinale roscoe against anticancer drug doxorubicin-induced acute nephrotoxicity* (Ajith, 2008)

244 *Ginger (Zingiber officinale) reduces acute chemotherapy-induced nausea: a URCC CCOP study of 576 patients* (Ryan, 2012)

245 *Ginger ingredients reduce viability of gastric cancer cells via distinct mechanisms.* (Ishiguro, 2007)

246 *Multiple mechanisms are involved in 6-gingerol-induced cell growth arrest and apoptosis in human colorectal cancer cells.* (S. H. Lee, 2008)

247 *Benefits of whole ginger extract in prostate cancer* (Karna, 2012)

248 *[6]-Gingerol, A Pungent Ingredient of Ginger, Inhibits Angiogenesis In Vitro and In Vivo* (Kim, 2005)

249 *Zerumbone, Sesquiterpene Photochemical From Ginger Inhibits Angiogenesis* (Park, 2015)

250 *Ginger Extract (Zingiber Officinale) has Anti-Cancer and Anti-Inflammatory Effects on Ethionine-Induced Hepatoma Rats* (Shafina Hanim Mohd Habib, 2008)

251 *Inhibitory Aromatase Effects of Flavonoids from Ginkgo Biloba Extracts on Estrogen Biosynthesis.*

estrogen-fueled cancers require suppression of estrogenic hormones to beat the cancer this may be an important option for many cancer patients. Estrogen-fueled cancers may include certain types of breast cancer, uterine cancer (a.k.a. endometrial cancer), ovarian cancer, certain types of prostate cancers, and certain types of colorectal cancer. Be sure to discuss your situation with your oncologist. In vitro studies have shown that ginkgo extract reverses chemotherapy resistance in gastric cancer cells. [252] One clinical trial involving thirty gastric cancer patients showed that oral intake of ginkgo exocarp polysaccharides resulted in the reduction of gastric tumors through growth inhibition and cancer cell death.[253] One particular clinical trial involving ginkgo's use against oxaliplatin-induced neuropathy showed that five out of six patients who used ginkgo after the second cycle of oxaliplatin therapy reported decreased intensity and duration of neuropathy.[254] Ginkgo contains a substance known as ginkgolic acid. Although some sources state that ginkgolic acid inhibits cancer through cell death[255] it is important to know that it is also a highly toxic substance which can also harm your healthy cells in like manner.[256] [257] According to one source *"Experiments performed by Professor Krieglstein, at the University of Pharmacology in Marburg revealed that ginkgolic acids display neurotoxic effects besides the fact that they are allergenic. With increasing concentrations of ginkgolic acids, you get a higher rate of cells death, up to more than 70 percent."*[258] If you choose to use ginkgo supplements I strongly urge you to avoid extracts which contain ginkgolic acid as the extracts are much more concentrated than the whole herb. Do not take any doses higher than your practitioner recommends. Dosage strength depends on your size, health, and which conditions you are being treated for. Consult with a competent practitioner before use. *Precautions: Ginkgo biloba has constituents which can effect CYP substrates* (see chapter 7 of this book) *so be careful to know which other medications you are taking before using this herb. Do not use ginkgo for at least 48 hours before surgery. Do not use if you have a history of seizures. Do not use if you are taking MAOI medications. Check with your prescribing physicians first to make sure other medications you are taking will not interact with ginkgo. May slightly increase the risk of some breast cancers. May cause changes in heartbeat.*

(Park, 2015)

252 *Ginkgo Biloba Extract Enhances Chemotherapy Sensitivity and Reverses Chemoresistance through suppression of the KSR1-mediated ERK1 / 2 Pathway in Gastric Cancer Cells* (Shi-Quan) Liu, 2015)

253 *Therapeutic Mechanism of Ginkgo Biloba Exocarp Polysaccharides on Gastric Cancer"*(Ai_Hua Xu, 2003)

254 *Ginkgo biloba (GB) Extract as a Neuroprotective Agent in Oxaliplatin (Ox)-induced Neuropathy.* (Marshall, 2004)

255 *Antitumor Effects of Ginkgolic Acid in Human Cancer Cell Occur Via Cell Cycle Arrest and Decrease the Bcl-2/Bax Ratio to Induce Apoptosis* (C. Zhou, 2010)

256 *Ginkgolic Acids Induce Neuronal Death and Activate Protein Phosphatase type-2c* (Ahlemeyer, 2001)

257 **Principles and Practice of Phytotherapy, Modern Herbal Medicine, 2,** (2013), p. 617, Kerry Bone, Simon Y. Mills

258 **Examining the Science Behind Nutraceuticals**, Proceedings of the AAPS Dietary Supplements Forum (2001) p.61

GLUTAMINE:

The amino acid known as glutamine, a.k.a. L-glutamine, has been shown to enhance the cancer-killing power of methotrexate,[259] protect the gastrointestinal system from chemotherapy symptoms, [260]protect patients from nerve damage caused by oxaliplatin treatments,[261] reduce the duration of chemotherapy induced diarrhea.[262] and reduce genetic damage caused by cisplatin therapy,[263] One study showed that a "glutamine cocktail" combining beta–hydroxy-beta-methylbutyrate (HMB), L-arginine and L-glutamine showed a significant reduction in cachexia.[264] The dosages of the cocktail ingredients used in the study were shown to be 1,000mg of HMB and 4,600mg each of 14g of L-arginine, together, three times daily (totaling 3g and 14g daily, respectively). For chemotherapy-induced mouth sores use glutamine suspension 4g as a swish and swallow therapy every four hours around the clock beginning with the first dose of chemotherapy until symptoms are resolved. *Precautions: Supplements may worsen existent liver disease. May cause a reaction in people sensitive to glutamates. Do not use if you have been diagnosed with mania disorders. Do not use if you have a history with seizures. May reduce the effectiveness of some chemotherapy agents – consult with your oncologist.* **Side note:** Though cancer cells use glutamine as a fuel source studies in humans have not found that glutamine supplements stimulate the growth of cancers in people undergoing chemotherapy.

GLUTATHIONE:

Glutathione is an antioxidant made by your liver using the amino acids glycine, glutamine and the sulfur-containing amino acid cysteine. Studies have shown that glutathione reduces the risk of neuropathy when undergoing chemotherapy with the platinum agents oxaliplatin[265] and cisplatin.[266] Your bodily reserves of glutathione can be depleted through poor diet, toxins, severe illness, and trauma. Dietary sources of glutathione include: Sulfurous vegetables such as garlic, onions, asparagus, and the brassica family,[267] as well as avocados, squash, and tomatoes. Eat these raw in order to retain the glutathione. Alternatively, you may purchase glutathione supplements which are usually labeled as acetyl-glutathione. Typical supplemental dosage is 10mg

259 *Effect of Glutamine on Methotrexate Efficacy and Toxicity* (Rubio, 1998)
260 *Clinical Trial: Prophylactic Intravenous Alanyl-glutamine Reduces the Severity of Gastrointestinal Toxicity Induced by Chemotherapy – A Randomized Crossover Study* (Y. Li, 2009)
261 *Oral Glutamine Is Effective For Preventing Oxaliplatin-induced Neuropathy in Colorectal Cancer Patients* (Wang, 2007)
262 *Glutamine for Chemotherapy Induced Diarrhea: A Meta-analysis.* (J. Sun, 2012)
263 *Pre-treatment With Glutamine Reduces Genetic Damage Due To Cancer Treatment With Cisplatin* (Oliveira, 2013)
264 *Reversal of Cancer-related wasting using oral supplementation with a combination of beta-hydroxy-beta – methylbutyrate, arginine, and glutamine.* (May, 2002);
265 *Neuroprotective effect of reduced glutathione on oxaliplatin-based chemotherapy in advanced colorectal cancer: a randomized, double-blind, placebo-controlled trial.* (Cascinu, 2002)
266 *Chemotherapy-induced peripheral neuropathy: Prevention and treatment strategies* (Wolf, 2008)
267 All cabbages, Arugula, bok choy, cauliflower, collard greens, broccoli, broccoli rabe, broccoli sprouts, Brussels sprouts, daikon, horseradish, kale, kohlrabi, komatsuna, mizuna, mustard greens, radishes, romanesco, rutabaga, tatsoi, turnips, turnip greens, wasabi, and watercress.

of glutathione per 1kg (2.2lbs) of body-weight. Therefore, a 68kg patient (150lbs) would take 750mg daily. Glutathione can be taken intravenously however this can only be done with your oncologist's recommendation. *Precautions: Inhaling glutathione may worsen asthma symptoms. May lighten skin tone.*

GRAPE SEED EXTRACT:

Do not confuse with grape*fruit* extracts. Studies using rat models have shown that grape seed extract may offer protection against heart damage,[268] liver damage,[269] and kidney damage[270] brought on by doxorubicin treatment. In vitro studies have shown grape seed extract to work synergistically with doxorubicin to inhibit both ER+ and ER- breast cancers.[271] One review of studies on grape seed extract found that the substance reduced cell growth *and* increased cell death in colorectal cancer, is toxic toward lung cancers , prostate cancer, oral squamous cells cancers and gastric adenocarcinomas, and had various methods of effects against different breast cancers (i.e. reduced metastasis, reduced tumor blood vessel formation, increase cancer cell death, etc. depending upon the specific type of cancer).[272] *Precautions: May thin the blood. Is high in antioxidants; talk to your oncologist to know whether these antioxidants may interfere with your current treatments. Ask your prescribing doctor before using this supplement if you have high blood pressure. May also interact with certain NSAID-type painkillers and heart medications. Side effects may include dizziness, headache, and nausea.*

GREEN TEA
Camellia sinensis

Green tea has many applications in holistic cancer management. In vitro tests have shown green tea to inhibit blood vessel formation in breast cancer cells and cause cell death in chronic lymphocytic leukemia (CLL) cells. One human trial involving 42 patients with early stage CLL observed that use of polyphenon-E, a green tea extract, resulted in a reduction in disease progression.[273] One study involving 41 patients with pre-cancerous lesions in the mouth observed a significantly lower rate of cancer development in patients taking the green tea supplements.[274] One in vivo study found that green tea extracts actually strengthens the efficacy of

---

268 *Cardioprotective Effects of Grape Seed Extract on Chronic Doxorubicin-induced Cardiac Toxicity in Wistar Rats* (Razmaraii, 2016)

269 *Efficacy of Grape Seed and Skin Extract Against Doxorubicin-induced oxidative stress in Rat Liver.* (Meherzia, 2015)

270 *Grape Seed and Skin Extract Protects Kidney from Doxorubicin-induced Oxidative Injury* (Meherzia, 2016).

271 *Synergistic Anti-cancer Effects of Grape Seed Extract and Conventional Cytotoxic Agent Doxorubicin Against Human Breast Carcinoma Cells* (Sharma, 2004)

272 *Anticancer and Cancer Chemopreventive Potential of Grape Seed Extract and Other Grape-based Products.* (Kuar, 2009)

273 *Phase II Trial of Daily, Oral, Polyphenon-E in Patients With Asymptomatic RAI Stage 0 to II Chronic Lymphocytic Leukemia* (Shanafelt, 2013)

274 *Phase II Randomized, Placebo-controlled Trial of Green Tea Extract in Patients with High-risk Oral Premalignant Lesions* (Tsao, 2009)

doxorubicin.[275] and can help protect a patient's heart from damage caused by doxorubicin.[276] Green tea has also been shown to increase the effectiveness of tamoxifen.[277] Some in vitro studies have found that green tea extract inhibits the growth of prostate cancer cells, however other constituents in green tea (and black tea) also tend to reduce the efficacy of some chemotherapy agents, especially those which are boron acid proteasome inhibitors, as the boronic acid binds with the EGCG[278] in green tea, rendering the drug ineffective. Therefore, do not use tea during active chemotherapy treatment cycles without speaking with your oncologist first. The University of Maryland Medical Center reports that using green tea triggered the activity of a certain gene that made prostate cancer cells less sensitive to the actions of chemotherapy drugs. Therefore it is better to take green tea supplements between prostate cancer chemotherapy cycles instead of during. *Precautions: May negatively interact with the chemotherapy agents such as irinotecan,[279] bortezomib,[280] and possibly other chemotherapy agents. Therefore, do not use green tea supplements during chemotherapy cycles. May increase the risk of breast cancer in post-menopausal women. May worsen peptic ulcers. May reduce the absorption of atropine-based medications. Do not use if you are taking MAOI antidepressants, lithium, atropine, iron, folic acid, verapamil, clozapine, ephedrine, contraceptive pills, and phenylpropanolamine. Whole green tea contains caffeine.*

GUARANA:
Paullinia cupana

This herb is a tropical plant native to Brazil which contains caffeine and is therefore popular as an energy booster. One study observed that this herb can help reduce cancer-related fatigue in breast cancer patients undergoing chemotherapy,[281] and a different study showed it can also help reduce mental fatigue.[282] Researchers have also found that guarana helps stabilize weight loss and increase appetite in patients with advanced cancers.[283] *Precautions: May cause heart rhythm disturbances and/or seizures in susceptible patients. May thin the blood. May increase blood pressure. May worsen glaucoma, diarrhea, irritable bowel syndrome, and bouts of anxiety. Do not take with other stimulant drugs such as cocaine, ephedrine, coffee, or*

275 *Modulation of Cancer Chemotherapy By Green Tea.* (Sadzuka, 1998)

276 *Effect of Green Tea Extract on Doxorubicin Induced Cardiovascular Abnormalities: Antioxidant Action* (Patil, 2011)

277 *The Combination of Green Tea and Tamoxifen is Effective Against Breast Cancer* (Sartippour, 2006)

278 Also known as *epigallocatechin gallate*

279 *Food-drug interaction of (-)-epigallocatechin-3-gallate on the pharmacokinetics of irinotecan and the metabolite SN-38.* (Lin, 2008)

280 *Green tea polyphenols block the anticancer effects of bortezomib and other boronic acid–based proteasome inhibitors.* (Encouse, 2009)

281 *Guarana (Paullinia cupana) Improves Fatigue in Breast Cancer Patients Undergoing Systemic Chemotherapy.* (de Oliveira Campos, 2011)

282 *Improved Cognitive Performance and Mental Fatigue Following a Multi-vitamin and Mineral Supplement with Added Guarana (Paullinia cupana).* (Kennedy, 2008)

283 *Guarana (Paullinia cupana) Improves Anorexia in Patients with Advanced Cancer.* (Palma, 2015)

amphetamines. May negatively interact with some antibiotics and other prescription medications. This herb is high in antioxidants.

HAOQIN QINGDAN:

This is a Traditional Chinese Medicine herbal formula which has been shown in animal studies to be protective of the liver during treatment with cyclophosphamide.[284] This formula contains the herbs sweet Annie (*artemisia annua*) and baikal skullcap (*Scutellaria baikalensis*). *Precautions: May cause allergic reaction. May depress the central nervous system so discontinue use two weeks before undergoing anesthesia. May lower blood sugar. May cause arrhythmias. Due to the potential for toxic side effects do not use this formula without professional oversight.*

HENNA:
Lawsonia inermis

Henna is small tree or shrub used for making an orange/red cosmetic dye used for decorating the hands, feet, and limbs. A small study involving nine cancer patients showed that patients treated with capecitabine began to experience relief from hand foot syndrome within 48 hours of topical henna application.[285] Just be aware that this substance may cause skin irritation or allergy in some patients. Henna artists (also known as mendhi artists) sometimes work at tattoo parlors but oftentimes own their own practice. If you cannot find a professional in your area you can make your own home made batch if you purchase henna powder from an Asia market, specialty store, or online; use package instructions to make your henna. Take note that some recipes also call for a squirt of lemon juice; omit this as it will sting when applied to the open areas on your skin. "Paint" a thin layer of the mix onto your affected areas and leave on for 15-20 minutes to dry. Cover the treated areas with gloves or socks and continue to leave the henna on for another 2 hours, then rinse off. Use at least once per week. *Precautions: Henna stains all surfaces it touches.. Some people may experience skin sensitivity or allergic reaction to henna. Never take henna by mouth. Never use black henna and do not accept black henna from a professional as it contains a coal tar dye that can cause blistering, open sores, and scarring.*

HOT PEPPERS:

Hot peppers contain a substance known as capsaicin, which gives the peppers their spicy flavor; the hotter the pepper, the more capsaicin it contains. It is well known in scientific circles that capsaicin reduces a neurotransmitter known as Substance P,[286] a compound which transmits pain signals and induces nausea.[287] Dosage: Normal dietary intake is safe. Because scientific studies have shown conflicting results as to whether capsaicin may be carcinogenic in high doses I do not

---

284 *The Hepatoprotective Effect of Haoqin Qingdan Decoction against Liver Injury Induced by a Chemotherapeutic Drug Cyclophosphamide* (Li, 2015)

285 *Topical Henna For Capecitabine Induced Hand-Foot Syndrome* (Yucel, 2008)

286 *Differential effects of capsaicin on the content of somatostatin, substance P, and neurotensin in the nervous system of the rat* (Gamse, 1981)

287 *Potential of Substance P Antagonists as Antiemetics* (Diemunsch, 2000)

recommend using oral capsaicin supplements without the oversight of an experienced practitioner. *Precautions: Do not use capsaicin cream or cayenne pepper on surgical sites, radiation sites, broken skin, mucous membranes, or get it in your eyes. Taking cayenne internally for long periods can reduce your liver's ability to process certain prescription medications. Excessive use of capsaicin internally may increase the risk of developing liver and stomach cancers. Capsaicin may thin the blood. Excessive internal use may irritate the intestinal tract. Wash hands thoroughly after using the fresh peppers or the topical remedies. Women with lobular breast cancer should moderate their intake due to an increased risk of metastasis to the stomach. Peppers are in the nightshade family; avoid use if you are allergic to other members of nightshade such as potatoes, tomatoes, eggplants, tomatillos, ground cherries, and goji berries.*

HYDROXYMETHYL-BUTYRATE:

Also known as beta–hydroxy-beta-methylbutyrate, or "HMB," this substance is created by your own body when metabolizing an amino acid known as leucine, therefore intake of leucine in your diet can be important. Food sources of leucine include: Parmesan cheese, tofu, soybeans, red meats, chicken, fish, nuts, seeds, and white beans. It is also sold as a nutritional supplement in forms such as HMB-FA and HMB-Ca /CaHMB. Studies have shown that supplementation with HMB reduces tumor growth and prevents cachexia,[288] with a *"usual dose"* of 3g (3,000mg)[289] [290] which should be ideally taken as 1g three times over the course of a day to maintain consistent blood levels. Is also an ingredient used in glutamine "cocktails" to ward off cachexia (see "Glutamine" in this chapter). Do not confuse HMB with GHB (gamma hydroxybutyrate). *Precautions: Full safety studies have not yet been performed therefore use extreme caution if you have liver or kidney disease. Safety for long-term usage has not been established as of this writing. Beware that some of the food sources in this listing should not be eaten if you are on MAOI medications.*

IRON

Sometimes cancer, or certain cancer treatments, can cause a patient to become deficient in red blood cells – a condition known as anemia. Anemia may cause you to feel tired, weak, or lightheaded and can cause changes in heart rhythm as well as headaches. In most cases the easiest way to increase your red blood cell numbers is to increase your intake of iron, an essential mineral necessary for the formation of healthy red blood cells. Although iron supplements can be bought over the counter I strongly advise that you do not use them without your doctor's oversight. This is because your body does not naturally rid itself of excess iron, which can result in iron

---

288 *Beta-hydroxy-beta-methylbutyrate Supplementation Reduces Tumor Growth and Tumor Cell Proliferation Ex Vivo and Prevents Cachexia in Walker 256 Tumor-bearing Rats by Modifying Nuclear Factor-KappaB Expression.* (Nunes, 2008)

289 *Beta–hydroxy-beta-methylbutyrate Supplementation in Health and Disease: a Systematic Review of Randomized Trials.* (Molfino, 2013)

290 *β-hydroxy-β-methylbutyrate (HMB) attenuates muscle and body weight loss in experimental cancer cachexia* (Zaira Aversa, 2011)

toxicity *and death* if left untreated. Too much iron in your blood is known as "hemochromatosis" – the only way to treat this condition is through controlled bloodletting under the supervision of a physician. In order to avoid iron toxicity it is better to take your iron supplements only with your doctor's advice. He or she will order blood tests in regular intervals to ensure you do not develop hemochromatosis. If your doctor allows you to add an iron supplement to your treatment you can improve your body's absorption of the mineral by taking your supplements with a beverage high in vitamin C such as orange juice.[291] Do not use grapefruit juice because certain enzymes within it may hinder the absorption of the iron. Alternatively you may choose to increase your iron through diet instead of supplements. Iron sourced from animal products (a.k.a. "heme iron") is more readily absorbed in the body than iron sourced from plants. If you follow a vegan diet be sure you use vitamin C to get maximum absorption, but you should also know that vitamins B12 and B9 (folate) also help your body to process iron for better absorption. Although many commercial vegan foods are already supplemented with B12 consider discussing with your doctor whether you should add these vitamin B supplements to your diet if you need an iron boost. Dietary sources of iron include fortified cereals, red meats, liver, clams, oysters, mussels, beef, sardines, lentils, beans, and dark green leafy vegetables. Whether you follow a vegan diet or not, take note that some nutrients and food items inhibit the absorption of iron so you should go easy on those items in your iron-containing meals. These inhibitory foods include:

- Calcium – inhibits 50% iron absorption[292]
- Tea – polyphenols inhibit 60% iron absorption
- Coffee – polyphenols inhibit 39% iron absorption
- Soy products – contains phytates which bind the iron
- Egg yolks – contain phosvitin, which binds the iron

At this point I need to make a special note regarding dark green leafy vegetables as these are a little more complicated when it comes to iron absorption. Although dark green leafy vegetables are high in iron they oftentimes also contain high amounts of calcium, which as you can see in the above list, is a known iron inhibitor. The dark green leafy vegetables highest in calcium are kale, mustard greens, cooked collard greens, cooked spinach and bok choy. Dark green leafy vegetables oftentimes also contain oxalic acid, a compound which binds with the the iron thus making iron absorption *even more* difficult. Since oxalic acid is water soluble you should lightly boiling the greens for 3 minutes, which will leach out about one third of the oxalic acid without sacrificing too many other nutrients. Due to the oxalic acid leaching into the water you should not use the leftover broth for other food usage; use the cooled broth to water your houseplants instead. *Precautions: Iron is not naturally excreted from the body, therefore excess iron buildup in the system can become fatal if left untreated. Never take iron supplements without your physician's oversight. The use of rosemary herb may decrease iron levels therefore be careful of use if you already have low red blood cell counts.*

---

291 *Interaction of vitamin C and iron.* (Lynch, 1980)
292 Therefore, do not use calcium-fortified orange juice or milk with your iron

LEMON BALM:
Melissa Officinalis:

Also known as bee balm, (do not confuse with the plant *Monarda didymus*, also known as bee balm). this member of the mint family is a time-tested sedative that has been supported in scientific studies.[293] Sometimes lemon balm is used in tandem with valerian or German chamomile but it can also be used alone. Topical use of the essential oil of lemon balm has been shown to be significantly effective against skin infections of the herpes simplex virus (chicken pox, shingles, genital herpes, etc.)[294] which may help cancer patients whose lowered immune systems allowed an infection to appear. *Tea:* Steep 2 tablespoons (30ml) of dried herb in one cup hot water for ten minutes. Strain and drink. Use up to four times per day. *Tincture:* Use up to 60 drops of tincture, in divided doses, per day (mixed in plain water). *Capsules:* Take up to 500mg of the dried or powdered herb three times per day. *Essential oil:* Use 12 drops of essential oil mixed with 2 tablespoons vegetable oil and apply to the herpes lesions. *Precautions: Internal use may increase the effect of alcohol, prescription sedative medications, and the sedative effect of seizure medications. Be cautious when using heavy machinery or driving until you know how this herb affects you. May cause dizziness, nausea, and wheezing in some people. May inhibit thyroid hormones. May worsen glaucoma and heart arrhythmias. May interact with SSRI antidepressants. Has antioxidant properties which may interfere with some chemotherapy agents. Topical use may cause allergic reaction in some individuals, therefore do not use if you are allergic to plants in the mint family.*

LICORICE ROOT:
Glycyrhizza Glabra

Licorice root is actually a rhizome; a stem which grows horizontally underground. This herb contains a flavonoid known as isoliquiritigenin, which in vitro studies have shown to be effective in reversing human breast cancer resistance to chemotherapy medications.[295] Another study, also performed in vitro mentions *"An **in vivo** study demonstrated that [isoliquiritigenin] could chemosensitize breast [cancer stem cells]... with little toxicity to normal tissues and mammary stem cells."*[296] Typical dosage of commercial supplements should not exceed 300mg daily for long term, over the counter use. Higher dosages must be under the supervision of a doctor, and for no more than four weeks at a time. *Dried root decoction:* Boil 1-2 teaspoon (5-10ml) of dried root in 1 ½ cups (360ml) of water for 15 minutes. Strain and drink. Take no more than two servings daily. *Licorice powder infusion:* Steep ½ to 1 teaspoon (7-15ml) of licorice powder into 1 cup (240ml) of hot water for fifteen

---

293 *Pilot trial of Melissa officinalis L. leaf extract in the treatment of volunteers suffering from mild-to-moderate anxiety disorders and sleep disturbances.* (Cases, 2011)

294 *Attachment and penetration of acyclovir-resistant herpes simplex virus are inhibited by Melissa officinalis extract.* (Astani, 2014)

295 *Micro-RNA 25 Regulates Chemoresistance-Associated Autophagy in Breast Cancer Cells, a Process Modulated by the Natural Autophagy Inducer Isoliquiritigenin* (Wang, 2014)

296 *Dietary Compound Isoliquiritigenin Targets GRP78 to Chemosensitize Breast Cancer Stem Cells Via β-catenin / ABCG2 Signaling* (Wang, 2014)

minutes and drink. Take up to two cups daily. *Tincture:* Place ½ – 1 teaspoon (7-15ml) of tincture into ½ cup (120ml) of water and drink. Use up to two time daily. *Precautions: Isoliquiritigenin may have estrogenic effect; use caution in cases of estrogen-dependent cancers. If your oncologist agrees that you should use this supplement be sure to buy from a reputable company. A constituent of licorice called glycyrrhizin may cause severe side effects; be sure to use deglycyrrhizinated licorice instead. Do not use licorice if you have heart disease, arrhythmias, kidney disease, or high blood pressure. May cause tiredness, missed periods, water retention, and low potassium. Do not use if you are taking blood thinners, digoxin, or diuretic medications. May cause too much sodium retention therefore be careful of your salt intake. Do not use licorice without competent professional guidance.*

MAGNESIUM:

Studies have shown that supplementation with this mineral may protect patients' kidneys from the toxic side effects of cisplatin, a platinum-based chemotherapy agent.[297] Magnesium helps by preventing the accumulation of platinum in the kidneys. Other platinum-based chemotherapy agents include carboplatin, oxaliplatin, and phenanthriplatin. Platinum-based medications may cause magnesium deficiencies in patients, therefore it is essential that you take any magnesium supplements prescribed by your oncologist. *Precautions: Do not take more than 350mg per day of magnesium for adults (the amounts naturally present in your foods and other supplements count towards this number as well). Too much magnesium may cause heart rhythm disturbances, low blood pressure, confusion, and death. May interact with antibiotics, diuretics, blood thinners, muscle relaxants, and blood pressure medications. Use caution if you have kidney failure. Supplementation may cause diarrhea.*

MARSHMALLOW ROOT:
Althaea officinalis

Marshmallow is a plant from which the soft white confection known as "marshmallow" originated. The plant has a white starchy root which contains a mucilage that coats and soothes the esophagus and stomach lining thus giving protection from stomach acids. Through the ages marshmallow has been known to help reverse some of the damage caused by stomach acids during bouts of heartburn. Because of its strong demulcent properties many patients are also directed to use a marshmallow infusion to help relieve mouth sores or soothe hand and foot syndrome. *Infusion:* Fill a jar ¼ of the way with pieces of marshmallow root and then fill the jar to the top with lukewarm purified water. Put the lid on the jar and let sit overnight. In the morning strain off the root pieces; you should have a thickened, yellowish liquid in the jar. Store in the refrigerator. You can use this liquid as a mouth rinse, as a topical application for hand and foot syndrome, or to drink to relieve heartburn. If using it for heartburn drink 1 cup (240ml) of the infusion up to twice daily. If you

---

297 *Magnesium protects against cisplatin-induced acute kidney injury by regulating platinum accumulation* (Solanki, 2014)

would rather use a commercially prepared version of this herb here are the following guidelines: *Tincture*: Place 35 drops in 1 cup (240ml) plain water once daily. *Capsules:* Take up to 6g in divided doses through the day. (1,000 mg = 1gram) *Precautions: May interfere with the absorption of some medications, therefore consume the marshmallow infusion several hours before or after taking your medications. May interfere with blood sugar control. Do not take if you are on lithium. The herb contains salicylic acid, the main ingredient in aspirin – do not use if you are allergic to aspirin or are currently using any kind of aspirin therapy or other substances which also contain salicylic acid.[298]*

MELATONIN:

Melatonin is a natural hormone released from yours pineal gland which is located in the brain. Because this hormone regulates sleep and your circadian rhythm it should be taken no earlier than one hour before your regular sleep time. One study found that adding melatonin with certain chemotherapy regimens increased patient survival and tumor regression rates compared to patients who did not receive melatonin.[299] Another study showed that patients receiving melatonin experienced reduced risks of bleeding problems, nerve damage, heart damage, certain types of mouth sores, and fatigue brought on by chemotherapy.[300] Other studies have shown melatonin to reduce heart damage in patients using doxorubicin,[301] increase survival rates in patients with metastasis to the brain while reducing cancer progression,[302] increase the survival time of patients being treated for metastatic non-small cell lung cancer,[303] boost the efficacy of capecitabine against pancreatic cancer,[304] and, when combined with antioxidants (vitamin E, vitamin C, glutathione and N-acetylcysteine) offers a level of protection against cisplatin-induced hearing loss.[305] Melatonin is also used in varying dosages for different health issues. For cancer, typical dosing for treatment of solid tumors is 10-40mg daily during chemotherapy, radiation, or interleukin-2 therapy. It is usual to begin your melatonin seven days before the beginning of your chemotherapy cycle and continue taking it until the cycle is

298 Salicylate herbs include: Black haw (*Viburnum prunifolium*), cramp bark (*Viburnum opulus*), marshmallow root (*althaea officinalis*), meadowsweet (*Filipendula ulmaria)*, sweet birch (*Betula lenta*), white birch (*Betula papyrifera*), white willow bark (*salix alba*), and wintergreen (*Gaultheria procumbens*). This is not a comprehensive list, consult with an experienced herbalist.

299 Chemotherapy regimens included the following: Cisplatin with etoposide *or* only gemcitabine for lung cancer; doxorubicin *or* mitoxantrone *or* paclitaxel for breast cancer; 5-FU with folinic acid for gastro-intestinal tumors; and 5-FU with cisplatin for head and neck cancers.

300*Decreased toxicity and increased efficacy of cancer chemotherapy using the pineal hormone melatonin in metastatic solid tumour patients with poor clinical status.* (Lissoni, 1999)

301 *Role of Exogenous Melatonin on Adriamycin-induced Changes in the Rat Heart.* (Aydemir, 2010)

302 *A Randomized Study With the Pineal Hormone Melatonin Versus Supportive Care Alone in Patients With Brain Metastases Due to Solid Neoplasms* (Lissoni, 1994)

303 *Five Years Survival in Metastatic Non-small Cell Lung Cancer Patients Treated With Chemotherapy Alone or Chemotherapy and Melatonin; A Randomized Trial.* (Lissoni, 2003)

304 *Improvement of Capecitabine Antitumoral Activity By Melatonin in Pancreatic Cancer* (Ruiz-Rabelo, 2011)

305 *Ototoxicity caused by cisplatin is ameliorated by melatonin and other antioxidants* (Lopez-Gonzalez, 2000)

finished. *Precautions: Melatonin is a hormone your body uses to induce sleep, therefore supplementation with this hormone may cause drowsiness and altered mental status. In some people it may also cause disorientation, rapid heartbeat, abdominal cramps, and headaches. May also alter estrogen levels. Do not use if you are currently taking Nifedipine. Melatonin may thin the blood.*

MILK THISTLE:
Silybum marianum

Silymarin is the therapeutic substance found in milk thistle plants and their seeds. Because the green plant parts may have estrogenic effect you should use supplements harvested only from the seeds if you have an estrogen-fueled cancer. The most efficient way to take milk thistle is by purchasing encapsulated extracts; whole herb or seed tea is not therapeutic because silymarin is not very water soluble. It is fat soluble though, with an absorption rate of 30-50% [306] therefore I recommend that if you have only the whole herb or seed available to you then it should be consumed with a a serving of heart-healthy fats such as what is found in vegetable oils and nuts. When using whole seed be sure you crush the seeds (1 ½ teaspoons of whole seed) before steeping in order to receive the full benefits of the silymarin. Take up to three cups of the tea per day. Studies have shown that silymarin is effective in protecting healthy kidneys from cell death caused by cisplatin,[307] enhances the effect of doxorubicin against breast cancer while also limiting its toxic side effects,[308] and, according to the American Cancer Society, protects the liver from chemotherapy induced damage. Studies have shown that silymarin is effective in inducing cancer cell death, reducing inflammation, suppressing the proliferation of breast cancer cells, inhibiting tumor blood vessel formation, inhibiting metastasis, and is protective of the heart and liver against the toxic effects of chemotherapy.[309] The seeds of this herb also contain silibinin and isosylibin, substances which have been shown to be also protective of nerve cells in laboratory cultures.[310] Safe dosage for commercial supplements is up to 420mg daily containing at least 70% silymarin. Follow package directions. *Precautions: At high doses silibinin can elevate the levels of bilirubin and liver enzymes; do not take more than the recommended dosage. Do not use if you are allergic to plants in the ragweed family. May lower blood sugar. May change cholesterol levels. May cause digestive upset. May cause rash. Do not use if you are taking anti-psychotics, blood thinners, Phenytoin/Dilantin, or hormones*

---

306 *Hepatoprotective and Antiviral Functions of Silymarin Components in Hepatitis C Virus Infection.* (Polyak, 2013)

307*Silymarin selectively protects human renal cells from cisplatin-induced cell death* (Ninsontia, 2011)

308 *The Role of Milk Thistle Extract in Breast Carcinoma Cell Line (MCF-7) Apoptosis With Doxorubicin* (Rastegar, 2013)

309 *Multitargeted Therapy of Cancer by Silymarin* (Ramasamy, 2008)

310*Neurotrophic and Neuroprotective Effects of Milk Thistle (Silybum marianum) on Neurons in Culture* (Kittur 2002)

OMEGA 3 FATTY ACIDS

Clinical trials using omega 3 fatty acids fish oils showed that intake of these fatty acids may reduce cachexia if patients begin taking it during the very early stages of condition[311] and can reverse chemo-resistance.[312] There is also evidence that omega 3's can preserve muscle mass when taken during a course of chemotherapy.[313] Dietary sources of Omega 3's include wild caught salmon, mackerel, sardines, walnuts, flaxseed,[314] chia seed, winter squash, hemp seeds, urad dal beans, leafy greens and some vegetable oils. Vegan sources may not be as easily absorbed in the body. Be aware that many vegan omega 3 products also contain omega **6** fatty acids which may induce inflammation and increase your risk of cachexia (see chapter 8, subheading "Inflammation Diet" for details regarding omega 6's). If you are concerned about this you may want to consider using a vegan omega 3 supplement which does not have omega 6's in it. When using supplements take 1,200mg of Omega 3's daily. For dietary intake eat at least three servings of fatty fish per week. Take note that omega 3's should only be used if there is an issue with cachexia, and only under the guidance of trained professionals, since these fatty acids have been observed to reduce the effectiveness of some chemotherapy agents by 50%![315] *Precautions: May thin blood. Do not exceed recommended dosage. Supplements may contain allergens such as soy or nuts. Do not use both supplements AND diet to increase your intake.*

PAPAYA
Carica Papaya

This tropical fruit contains an abundance of papain, an enzyme which helps you digest food better – especially proteins – and can help stimulate the appetite. It is also known for reducing pain and inflammation. You can either eat the fresh fruit or purchase commercial supplements of this enzyme. Typical supplemental dosage is about 1500mg (1.5g) daily. *Precautions: Patients allergic to kiwi or figs may also be allergic to papaya or papain supplements. Supplements may cause damage to the throat membranes when taken in excessive doses. Papain thins the blood.*

QUERCETIN:

Quercetin is a fat soluble substance found in capers, onions, cranberries, plums, blueberries, cherries, apples, red leaf lettuce, and asparagus. One study observed that quercetin can inhibit the growth of glioma brain cancer cells[316] According to a report by News Medical Life Sciences, (August 5, 2009) "*In low concentrations quercetin behaves as an antioxidant, yet at high concentrations it*

---

311 *British Journal of Cancer*, 2011, Vol. 105, pp.1469-1473, "*Influence of Eicosapentaenoic Acid Supplementation on Lean Body Mass in Cancer Cachexia*" R. A. Murphy, et al

312 *Inhibition of Proliferation by Omega 3 Fatty Acids in Chemoresistant Pancreatic Cancer Cells* (Hering, 2007)

313 *Omega-3 fatty acids in cancer* (Laviano, 2013)

314 Whole flax seeds pass through your digestive system unchanged. You get more benefit from using ground flaxseed instead.

315 *Netherlands Cancer Institute*, "*New evidence for chemoresistance after consuming fish oil or fatty fish.*"(April 3, 2015) Based on the research of Dr. Emile Voest.

316 *Antiproliferative Effect of Quercetin in the Human U138MG Glioma Cell Line* (Braganhol, 2006)

becomes a cell damaging pro-oxidant." This pro-oxidant feature has shown quercetin to be useful in sensitizing melanoma and glioblastoma cancers to both chemotherapy and radiation. Several studies found quercetin acts synergistically to enhance agents such as doxorubicin,[317] cisplatin,[318] temozolomide,[319] dexamethasone,[320] vincristine,[321] 5-FU,[322] and etoposide.[323] Quercetin also protects the patient from the toxic effects of certain chemotherapy agents. For example, it helps reduce liver damage caused by doxorubicin and kidney damage caused by platinum agents. Other studies have shown that combining quercetin with other natural agents may also enhance the effect of certain chemotherapy treatments. For example, combining quercetin with thymoquinone, a substance from thyme plants and black cumin seed, along with cisplatin therapy gave much better results than cisplatin alone.[324] [325] Combining quercetin with the polyphenol resveratrol may reduce bone marrow damage during etoposide treatments.[326] In vitro studies have shown that quercetin can reverse chemo-resistance to doxorubicin [327] and other chemo agents.[328] Because quercetin is fat soluble you should take your supplements or quercetin-rich foods with heart healthy fats such nuts, peanuts, seeds, and vegetable oils. *Precautions: Do not take quercetin if you are taking cyclosporine, felodepine, or nifedipine. May decrease the effect of some antibiotics. May increase estrogen levels. When combined with resveratrol, be aware that resveratrol is known to thin the blood.*

RESVERATROL:

This is an anti-cancer polyphenol compound found in several plant sources

---

317 *Quercetin Potentiates Doxorubicin Mediated Antitumor Effects Against Liver Cancer Through p53/Bcl-xl.* (Wang, 2012)

318 *Quercetin-induced Inhibition and Synergistic Activity With Cisplatin – A Chemotherapeutic Strategy for Nasopharyngeal Carcinoma Cells* (Daker, 2012)

319 2011, *Kinetic Studies of the Effects of Temodal and quercetin an astrocytoma cells.* (Jakubowicz-Gil, 2011)

320 *Quercetin Displays Anti-myeloma Activity and Synergistic Effect with Dexamethasone in Vitro and in Vivo Xenograft Models* (Xing Guo, 2015)

321 *Simultaneous Liposomal Delivery of Quercetin and Vincristine for Enhanced Estrogen Receptor-negative Breast Cancer Treatment* (Wong, 2010)

322 *Quercetin Induces Apoptosis and Enhances 5-FU Therapeutic Efficacy in Hepatocellular Carcinoma* (Dai, 2016)

323 *Effects of Quercetin on the Pharmacokinetics of Etoposide After Oral or Intravenous Administration of Etoposide in Rats.* (Li, 2009)

324 *Synergism from Combinations of Cisplatin and Oxaliplatin with Quercetin and Thymoquinone in Human Ovarian Tumour Models* (Nessa, 2011)

325 This study found that using the quercetin and thymoquinone two hours before the platinum agents were administered gave the best results.

326 *Modulatory Effect of Quercetin on DNA Damage, Induced by Etoposide in Bone Marrow Cells and on Changes in the Activity of Antioxidant Enzymes in Rats* (Cierniak, 2004)

327 *Quercetin potentiates the effect of adriamycin in a multidrug-resistant MCF-7 human breast-cancer cell line: P-glycoprotein as a possible target.* (Scambia, 1994)

328 *Quercetin Suppresses Drug-Resistant Spheres via the p38 MAPK–Hsp27 Apoptotic Pathway in Oral Cancer Cells* (Chen, 2012); *Abstract 5560: Quercetin overcomes chemotherapy resistance in triple negative breast cancer* (Srinivasan, 2015)

such as red wine, red grapes, dark chocolate,[329] peanut skins and blueberries. Research from in vitro and in vivo studies has found that resveratrol can be effective in re-sensitizing cancers to several kinds of chemotherapy medications[330] and is also protective of patients' kidneys during chemotherapy treatments.[331] Although low doses of resveratrol has shown to be protective against cisplatin-induced hearing loss, higher doses of the substance proved to do further harm.[332] Resveratrol may be poorly absorbed by the body so I advise you to speak to your physician or practitioner as to whether you should use a higher potency commercial supplement. *Precautions: Drink red wine in moderation (1-2 servings daily) as too much alcohol may encourage breast cancer. Resveratrol may thin the blood. May have estrogenic effect.*

ROMAN CHAMOMILE:
Anthemis nobilis / Chamaemelum nobile

Do not confuse with German chamomile (*Matricaria chamomilla*). Chamomiles are commonly known to have tranquilizing effects and promote sleep. This sedation is thought to be due to the presence of apigenin, a substance in the plant which binds to the same receptors in the brain[333] that are affected by prescription sedatives such as Valium.[334] When using chamomile as an aromatherapy agent take note: Although German chamomile and Roman chamomile both give sedative and anti-inflammatory effects when orally consumed, their levels of healing agents are not matched. Therefore, Roman chamomile essential oils used in aromatherapy is a better calming agent and German chamomile oil is better as a topical agent against inflammation.

ROSEMARY:
Rosemarinus officinalis

Rosemary is an evergreen plant commonly used as a culinary flavoring. One report states that in vitro studies show rosemary extracts can inhibit the growth of colon cancer as well as enhance the activity of the chemotherapy agents 5-fluorouracil, trastuzumab, tamoxifen, and paclitaxel and reverse resistance to cisplatin. This report also notes that when rosemary is combined with vitamin D analogues against acute myeloid leukemia it enhances the therapeutic effect. This report also covered information from in vivo studies, which observed the reduction of human colon cancer tumors in mice. The report noted that the levels of rosemary needed for use in human treatment would require concentrated extracts, as whole herb intake would not be sufficient.[335] For aromatherapy treatments, clinical studies have

---

329 Natural process dark chocolate has a significantly higher amount of antioxidants and polyphenols (such as resveratrol) than dutch process chocolate or milk chocolate.

330 *Chemosensitization of Tumors by Resveratrol* (Gupta, 2011)

331 *Chemosensitizing and Nephroprotective Effect of Resveratrol in Cisplatin-treated Animals* (Osman, 2015)

332 *Molecular Mechanisms of Protective Effect of Resveratrol Against Cisplatinium Induced Ototoxicity* (Olgun, 2013)

333 Specifically, the benzodiazepine receptors.

334 Chamomile: A herbal medicine of the past with bright future. (Srivastava, 2010)

335 *Anticancer Effects of Rosemary (Rosmarinus officinalis L.) Extract and Rosemary Extract Polyphenols.* (Moore, 2016)

confirmed that inhalation of the essential oil of rosemary causes a physically stimulating response by increasing brain wave activity, blood pressures and heart rates; participants reported feeling energized and refreshed.[336] *Precautions: Do not use rosemary oil internally. Do not use if you have a seizure disorder or are taking diuretics. May thin the blood. May interfere with ACE inhibitors. May cause buildup of lithium medications.*

SEAWEED:

Some chemotherapy medications give you an unappetizing metallic taste in your mouth. You could try counteracting that taste by eating foods with seaweed in them such as laverbread, mi yuk guk, miso soup, seaweed chips, etc.

SELENIUM:

Selenium is a dietary mineral found in foods such as Brazil nuts, garlic, oysters, tuna, sunflower seeds, whole wheat breads, shiitake mushrooms, white button mushrooms, chia seeds, brown rice,and broccoli. Since the adult daily requirement of selenium is 50mcg daily, take note that Brazil nuts in particular have a reputation for being very high in selenium (400mcg per ounce!), therefore you should be sure you do not over-indulge so as to avoid selenium toxicity. Taking vitamin E with selenium helps with selenium absorption. There are different forms of selenium: L-selenomethionine, selenium-methyl-L-selenocysteine and sodium selenite.[337] L-selenomethionine induces cell death only in cancer cells which still have a working p53 gene (the apoptosis/cancer cell suicide gene), whereas selenium-methyl L-selenocysteine induces apoptosis in cancer cells which have no working p53 gene. As for sodium selenite, this increases expression of the enzyme glutathione peroxidase – an antioxidant substance, helping to prevent cancer from developing. Although it isn't necessarily wrong to use just one form of the mineral it is better to use all forms because individual cancer cells, even within the same tumor, may or may not have working p53 genes, thus using all forms will target things all the way around. The best way to get all forms is to consume the food sources instead of simply relying on commercial supplements (which tend to feature only one form of selenium). Some people may bring up the fact that one particular study published in 2009, known as "SELECT," appeared to show that selenium had no effect on cancer[338] and therefore they do not put any faith in the mineral. Since the vast majority of scientific evidence shows selenium to be effective against cancer, what happened for this study to be contrary? Unfortunately, this study used only *one* form of selenium combined with synthetic vitamin E which forces out natural vitamin E in your body cells.[339] (see the subheading "Vitamin E" in this chapter). The use of only one form of selenium along

---

336 *Effects of Inhaled Rosemary Oil On Subjective Feelings and Activities of the Nervous System.* (Sayorwan, 2013)

337 Also known as selenium monomethionine.

338 *Effect of selenium and vitamin E on risk of prostate cancer and other cancers: the Selenium and Vitamin E Cancer Prevention Trial (SELECT).* (Lippman, 2009)

339 *Gamma-tocopherol traps mutagenic electrophiles such as NO(X) and complements alpha-tocopherol: physiological implications.* (Christen, 1997)

with the use of a non-natural vitamin E was enough to affect the outcome of the study. In truth, the majority of research has shown selenium to be very effective against cancer. One study showed that selenium supplementation enhanced the anti-cancer effects of both doxorubicin and paclitaxel.[340] Another study observed that women with ovarian cancer who supplemented with 200mcg of selenium daily experienced reduced side effects (hair loss, weakness, loss of appetite) caused by chemotherapy agents as well as saw increased levels of white blood cells.[341] Other studies showed selenium to provide some protection from nerve damage caused by cisplatin therapy [342] as well as protection from kidney damage and bone marrow damage from cisplatin therapy.[343] *Precautions: Taking doses above 400 mcg daily can cause toxicity. High doses may interfere with vitamin C absorption. Selenium supplementation in men with prostate cancer may increase risk of cancer death; therefore men with prostate cancer should not take selenium supplements without discussing it with their oncologists first. Do not supplement if you have an autoimmune disorder or have had an organ transplant. Supplements may negatively affect under-active thyroids. May increase risk of excessive bleeding during surgery so discontinue use two weeks before. May interact with blood thinners, cholesterol reducers, or niacin therapy. May increase the action of sedatives.*

SOLUBLE FIBER:

Soluble fiber is a food substance which helps absorb water in the intestines, thereby decreasing problems with diarrhea and decreasing problems with constipation. Foods which contain soluble fiber include: Dry beans, peas, lentils, oatmeal, oat bran, Brussels sprouts, and flax seeds. Because flax seeds pass through the digestive system when used whole they should be ground before consuming. *Precautions: Do not overdo your intake of soluble fiber as it may interfere with the absorption of other nutrients or medications.*

ST. JOHN'S WORT:

Hypericum perforatum

Also known as goatweed, the therapeutic substances in St. John's Wort (SJW) are easily damaged by heat and light, therefore it is advisable to store your SJW products in a dark container away from direct heat and light sources. Although SJW is commonly known for addressing clinical depression its active constituent, hyperforin, also has value when it comes to cancer therapies. One study observed that hyperforin and another substance in SJW known as aristoforin, induce cell death and inhibit tumor blood vessel formation in cancerous tumors.[344] A different study tested

---

340 *Effect of Selenium in Combination with Adriamycin or Taxol on Several Different Cancer Cells* (Vadgama, 2000)

341 *Selenium as an element in the treatment of ovarian cancer in women receiving chemotherapy.* (Sieja, 2004)

342 *Selenium Partially Prevents Cisplatin-induced Neurotoxicity: A Preliminary Study* (Erken, 2014)

343 *The Protective Role of Selenium on the Toxicity of Cisplatin-contained Chemotherapy Regimen in Cancer Patients* (Hu, 1997)

344 *Hyperforin and Aristoforin Inhibit Lymphatic Endothelial Cell Proliferation In Vitro an Suppress*

the effects of hypericin, another substance in SJW, in 42 patients with recurrent brain tumors. Patients took oral doses[345] of synthetic hypericin once each morning for three months. According to the study, 20% of the patients with glioblastoma multiforme tumors responded to treatment and 29% of patients with anaplastic astrocytoma tumors responded.[346] However, one must be careful when using this along with chemotherapy treatments because numerous studies have shown SJW significantly interferes with the activity of many chemotherapy agents. The effects of SJW may continue for up to four weeks after discontinuing use, therefore you must stop using SJW at least four weeks before starting your affected chemotherapy treatments. If you are already using SJW for depression you need to speak to your prescribing doctor about switching to another antidepressant for the duration of your cancer treatments. Due to its reputation to interact with so many other medications take this herb only under the supervision of a physician. *Precautions: Strongly interacts with several medications and herbs. May interfere with the absorption of essential minerals. May cause increased skin sensitivity to radiation treatments or sunlight. Discontinue use at four weeks before and one week after chemotherapy treatment cycles. May cause headache, dry mouth, or sleepiness. Do not use if you've had an organ transplant. Do not use for at least two weeks before undergoing general anesthesia. May cause nerve pain in some patients. May decrease libido. Excessive use may result in withdrawal symptoms when suddenly stopped.*

SWEET ANNIE:
Artemisia annua

This herb goes by other names such as Chinese wormwood, sweet wormwood, sweet sagewort, and sweet mugwort. Sweet Annie contains a substance known as artemisinin which is commonly known for its anti-malarial properties but has been shown to be an effective treatment against many types of cancer cells. Studies have observed that the combined use of Sweet Annie with iron can kill up to 98% of cancer cells within a mere sixteen hours without harming most healthy cells[347] and that the herb is also effective in reducing the size of neuroblastoma brain tumors.[348] One review of studies noted that artemisinin could inhibit cancer in multiple ways including the inducement of cell death, inhibition of tumor blood vessel formation, disruption of cancer cell movement, and cessation of cancer cell cycles.[349] A double-case study published in 2005 reporting on two patients with metastasized melanomas observed that artesunate, a substance derived from artemisinin, boosted the effectiveness of the chemotherapy agent fotemustine in one patient and halted the progression of metastasis to the lungs and spleen in the second patient. The second patient, who was using the chemotherapy agent dacarbazine, was also noted to have a

---

Tumor-induced Lymphangiogenesis In Vivo. (Rothley, 2009)

345 Dosages ranged from .05 -0.50mg of hypericin per kg of patient body weight

346 *A Phase 1 /2 Study of Orally Administered Synthetic Hypericin for Treatment of Recurrent Malignant Gliomas.* (Couldwell, 2011)

347 *Effects of artemisinin-tagged holotransferrin on cancer cells.* (Lai, 2005)

348 *Artemisinin reduces cell proliferation and induces apoptosis in neuroblastoma.* (Zhu, 2014)

349 *Anticancer activities of artemisinin and its bioactive derivatives* (Firestone, 2009)

survival rate of 4 years whereas normally a patient in that situation would have an average survival of only 2-5 *months*.[350] Another case study involving a patient with laryngeal squamous cell cancer (a tumor on his vocal cords) observed that a specific treatment regimen which included both injections and oral administration of artesunate on a daily basis resulted in a 70% reduction in the size of the tumor.[351] Artesunate has also been observed to inhibit tumor blood vessel formation through suppression of VEGF.[352] *Precautions: Do not use Sweet Annie if you have a history of seizures. Topical preparations using this herb may cause skin rash. May cause dizziness, do not drive. May cause nausea. Do not use if you have stomach ulcers or other digestive issues. Do not use if you are allergic to plants in the ragweed family. May cause liver problems in susceptible patients. Over-use of the herb may cause resistance; use with competent professional supervision.*

SWEET BEE VENOM:

Since this is actually made from the venom of honeybees this is not a treatment for those who are allergic to bee stings or those who are trying to maintain a vegan lifestyle. In one case series it was observed that a seven day course of treatment with sweet bee venom in five patients showed improvement in neuropathy symptoms without side effects.[353] In a different case series researchers treated 11 patients with sweet bee venom for three weeks, showing significant improvement in pain and neuropathy scales.[354] *Precautions: Do not use if you are allergic to bee venom. Vegans should know that bee venom also goes by the names apitoxin and mixed vespids. Allergies may occur in patients who had no previous allergy to the venom. Do not use without the oversight of a physician.*

TAMALAKI:

Phyllanthus Fraternus

In vivo studies have shown that this tropical African plant may protect both the liver and the kidneys from cyclophosphamide treatment.[355] [356] Another study, using rat models, noted that using tamalaki in conjunction with the combination of cisplatin *and* cyclophosphamide helped reduce the toxicity of the agents without reducing their efficacy.[357] Commercial preparations of this herb are sometimes mixed

---

350 *Artesunate in the treatment of metastatic uveal melanoma--first experiences.* (Berger, 2005)

351 *Case Report of a Laryngeal Squamous Cell Carcinoma Treated with Artesunate.* (Singh, 2002)

352 Inhibitory effects of artesunate on angiogenesis and on expressions of vascular endothelial growth factor and VEGF receptor KDR/flk-1. (Chen, 2004)

353 *Effects of Sweet Bee Venom Pharmacopuncture Treatment for Chemotherapy-induced Peripheral Neuropathy: A Case Series.* (Park, 2011).

354 *Sweet Bee Venom Pharmacopuncture for Chemotherapy-induced Peripheral Neuropathy.* (Yoon, 2012)

355 *Evaluation of the antioxidant and hepatoprotective effect of Phyllanthus fraternus against a chemotherapeutic drug cyclophosphamide* (Lata, 2014)

356 *Protective effect of Phyllanthus fraternus against cyclophosphamide-induced nephrotoxicity in rats*

(Moirangthem, 2017)

357 *Protective Effect of Phyllanthus Fraternus Against Mitochondrial Dysfunction Induced by Co-*

with other plants in the *phyllanthus* family; be sure you are buying from a reputable company that is giving you a pure product. Use this herb only under the supervision of your doctor and a competent practitioner. *Precautions: As of this writing little is known about the safety of long-term use of this herb. May increase the effects of diabetic and blood pressure medications.*

THYMOQUINONE:
(See also "Black Cumin" in this chapter)

Thymoquinone is an antioxidant found in plants such as black cumin (*Nigella Sativa,/N. cretica*), bee balm (M*onarda fistulosa /M. didyma*) and common thyme (*Thymus vulgaris*). In vivo studies have shown that thymoquinone is effective in protecting the liver from the damage caused by the chemotherapy medication tamoxifen,[358] inhibits the proliferation of Er+ / PR+ breast cancer cells,[359] as well as inhibiting the proliferation of numerous other forms of cancer.[360] A phase 1 clinical trial involving patients with advanced cancers showed no toxic side effects of using up to 2,600mg of thymoquinone daily.[361] *Precautions: Black cumin may lower blood sugar, lower blood pressure, and slow your blood clotting response. Do not use thyme if you are allergic to oregano. May have blood thinning effect. Thyme may have estrogenic effect. May interact with blood thinning medications.*

VALERIAN ROOT:
Valeriana officinalis

The valepotriates contained in valerian root have a sedative effect that's been known through the centuries. Many patients prefer to use valerian instead of prescription sleep aids because the herb does not carry side effects such as daytime grogginess, dizziness, tremors, etc. Some physicians believe valerian interferes with chemotherapy treatments due to animal studies showing valerian to increase the CYP enzymes which metabolize drugs, however one small study involving twelve healthy volunteers noted that the use of valerian had very little effect on CYP activity,[362] and a second study of twelve other healthy volunteers published the following year also noted that the use of valerian root had no significant impact on CYP metabolism.[363] Therefore you should speak with your prescribing physician(s) before deciding whether to use this herb. Typical dosage is one capsule, 450-500mg strength, one hour before bedtime. Supplements should be made from valerian root standardized to

---

administration of Cisplatin and Cyclophosphamide. (Kumari, 2011)

358 *Protective role of thymoquinone against liver damage induced by tamoxifen in female rats* (Suddek, 2014)

359 *Cellular Responses with Thymoquinone Treatment in Human Breast Cancer Cell Line MCF-7.* (Motaghed, 2013)

360 *Review on Molecular and Therapeutic Potential of Thymoquinone in Cancer.* (Banerjee, 2014).

361 *Phase 1 Safety and Clinical Activity Study of Thymoquinone in Patients With Advanced Refractory Malignant Disease* (Al-Amri, 2009)

362 *Multiple Night Time Doses of Valerian (Valeriana officinalis) Had Minimal Effects on CYP3A4 activity and No Effect on CYP2D6 Activity in Healthy Volunteers.* (Donovan, 2004)

363 *In Vivo Effects of Goldenseal, Kava Kava, Black Cohosh, and Valerian on Human Cytochrome P450 1A2, 2D6, 2E1, and 3A4.5 Phenotypes.* (Gurley, 2005)

0.8 -1% valerenic acid. Do not take for longer than four weeks. *Precautions: Valerian should be discontinued at least one week before surgery. Be careful about using alcohol, heavy machinery or driving until you know how the herb affects you. Do not use if you have liver or pancreas problems. May interact negatively with certain prescription medications so consult with your physician before use.*

VITAMINS B6 & B12 COMBINED:

Studies have shown that the combination of B6 (up to 200mg daily) and B12 (1000mcg daily) may reduce the risk of developing chemotherapy-induced neuropathy.[364] Please note that sources state that B6 treatment is dose dependent: Doses of vitamin B6 from 50 – 200 mg are shown to be effective, however it was observed that doses higher than 200mg actually promoted neuropathy. Also note that the dose for B12 is <u>micro</u>grams, not milligrams. Dietary vitamin B12 is primarily sourced from animal-based products and fortified vegan products: Some studies have shown that a deficiency in vitamin B12 may be a factor in acquiring nerve damage[365] and other studies have shown that the combination of B6 and B12 therapy may reduce the risk of chemotherapy-induced nerve damage. Another study involving 64 patients with malignant pleural mesothelioma being treated with pemetrexed found that the patients who were supplemented with vitamin B12 and folic acid tolerated the treatments better and had, on average, a 5 month longer survival span.[366] Speak with your doctor to decide which dosage of vitamin B12 you should be taking. *Precautions: Do not take B12 if you have Leber's Disease. B12 may interact with Chloramphenicol. Do not use supplements if you have developed ischemic heart disease.[367] B vitamins may interact with Parkinson's medications, seizure medications, or Cordarone. Avoid supplementing with B12 if you had recent insertion of a heart stent.*

VITAMIN C:

Although studies have not shown that oral intake of vitamin C is useful against cancer it has been shown that intravenous use of the vitamin may be beneficial. One study published in 2014 states *"There is consistent evidence that [intravenous] vitamin C can improve cancer patients' quality of life and decrease multiple aspects of fatigue."*[368] Earlier that year a single case study was published which showed that a patient with recurrent breast cancer experienced improvement in fatigue after being treated with 50g of intravenous vitamin C twice weekly.[369] These support an earlier study which showed intravenous vitamin C to improve the quality

---

364 *Vitamins B6 and B12 Supplementation to Prevent Chemotherapy-Induced Neuropathy: Interim Analysis of the Taxane Cohort* (Verschraegen, 2009)

365 *Chemotherapy-Induced Peripheral Neuropathy (CIPN) and Vitamin B12 Deficiency* (Schloss, 2015)

366 *Phase II Study of Pemetrexed with and without Folic Acid and Vitamin B 12 as Front-line Therapy in Malignant Pleural Mesothelioma.* (Scagliotti, 2003)

367 *Cancer Incidence and Mortality after Treatment with Folic Acid and Vitamin B 12* (Ebbing, 2009)

368 *The Effect of Intravenous Vitamin C on Cancer- and Chemotherapy-Related Fatigue and Quality of Life* (Carr, 2014)

369 *Relief from cancer chemotherapy side effects with pharmacologic vitamin C* (Carr, 2014)

of life in breast cancer patients.[370] Intravenous vitamin C cannot be bought over the counter. You must have a properly licensed professional to administer this therapy. *Precautions: Do not use excessive amounts of oral vitamin C supplements as a substitute for intravenous vitamin C as this will cause severe diarrhea, abdominal cramping, and nausea.*

VITAMIN E:
Tocopherols

Vitamin E, a fat soluble vitamin, is known for its excellent antioxidant and cancer fighting properties, however it is important to know that not all forms of vitamin E are equal. The most common form in commercial supplements is known as alpha tocopherol, however it is also important to get plenty of another form, known as gamma tocopherol. Food sources of gamma tocopherol include nuts, seeds, and vegetable oils. Although both alpha and gamma-tocopherol have shown to be effective in reducing heart disease and certain cancers, the gamma-tocopherol version has been shown be significantly more effective at removing the inflammation-causing nitrogen oxides[371] which contribute to the formation of cancer.[372] Gamma-tocopherol has also been observed to have inhibitive effects on prostate and lung cancers.[373] *Precautions: Vitamin E is a known blood thinner. Taking more than 300IU of this vitamin every day may increase the chance of hemorrhagic stroke by 22%. High doses may also cause nausea, diarrhea, and rash. Vitamin E supplementation immediately before and after angioplasty procedures is associated with delayed healing. May increase the risk of heart failure in diabetics. May increase the recurrence of head and neck cancers and may worsen prostate cancer. May interact with certain prescription medications. May decrease the benefits of niacin (vitamin B3) supplementation.*

WHEATGRASS:
Triticum aestivum

Do not confuse with *Thinopyrum intermedium*, which is another plant known as "wheatgrass." *Triticum aestivum* is prepared from the cotyledons (first leaves from the seedlings) of wheat plants. Wheatgrass that is harvested before the plant goes to seed is gluten free. Because wheatgrass is rather tough and hard to digest you will usually find it sold as a powder; it has a strong, grassy flavor. One pilot study observed that breast cancer patients receiving 2 ounces of wheatgrass juice (60 ml) daily experienced less problems with chemotherapy-induced side effects (such as

---

370 *Intravenous Vitamin C Administration Improves Quality of Life in Breast Cancer Patients during Chemo-/Radiotherapy and Aftercare: Results of a Retrospective, Multicentre, Epidemiological Cohort Study in Germany* (Vollbracht, 2011)

371 These can be found in places such as car exhaust and cigarette smoke.

372 *Gamma-tocopherol detoxification of nitrogen dioxide: superiority to alpha-tocopherol.* (Cooney, 1993)

373 *Gamma-tocopherol Induces Apoptosis in Androgen-responsive LNCaP Prostate Cancer Cells Via Caspase-dependent and Independent Mechanisms.* (Jiang 2004)

lowered blood counts) than patients who did not receive the wheatgrass.[374] In a preliminary trial, taking 2 ounces of wheatgrass per day during chemotherapy reduced the incidence of certain chemotherapy-related side effects (including anemia and a decline in white blood cell counts) in women with breast cancer. Taking wheatgrass did not appear to interfere with the anticancer effect of the chemotherapy. The chemotherapy used in this study was a combination of 5-fluorouracil, doxorubicin, and cyclophosphamide.[375] *Precautions: Raw wheatgrass may contain harmful microbes, depending upon the conditions in which it was harvested.*

WHITE WILLOW BARK:
Salix alba

White willow contains salicin, a substance that is converted into salicylic acid in your body, which is the active ingredient in aspirin.[376] To create this naturally at home mix 1 tablespoon of white vinegar (which contains acetic acid) into 1 cup of willow bark tea (3g of whole bark will contain 120mg of salicin). To make the tea: Add two teaspoons of willow bark to 10 ounces boiling water. Continue boiling for 10 minutes. Turn off the heat, strain out the bark pieces, cool the tea and drink. Do not drink more than three cups per day without competent professional oversight. If using commercial supplements go by package instructions. *Precautions: Do not use if you are allergic to aspirin. This herb is a blood thinner. Take caution if you are using other supplements which also contain salicylic acids.[377] Do not use if you are sensitive to salicylates such as aspirin, black haw (Viburnum prunifolium), cramp bark (Viburnum opulus), marshmallow root (althaea officinalis), meadowsweet (Filipendula ulmaria), sweet birch (Betula lenta), white birch (Betula papyrifera), and wintergreen (Gaultheria procumbens). This is not a comprehensive list, consult with an experienced herbalist.*

YELLOW DOCK:
Rumex crispus

Also known as curly dock, this herb's root is naturally high in iron. Due to the presence of oxalates in the green parts of the plant I advise using preparations made only from the root. Be sure to seek professional advice before using yellow dock supplements due to risk of accumulating too much iron in your system. *Precautions: This herb has a laxative effect. It can also cause blood to clot more easily, so use caution if you are at risk. Do not use if you are allergic to plants in the ragweed family. Do not use if you have digestive ulcers or blockages. Do not use if you are at*

---

374 *Wheatgrass Juice May Improve Hematological Toxicity Related to Chemotherapy in Breast Cancer Patients: a Pilot Study* (Bar-Sela, 2007)

375 *Wheatgrass juice may improve hematological toxicity related to chemotherapy in breast cancer patients: a pilot study* (Bar-Sela, 2007)

376 Aspirin's active ingredient is acetylsalicylic acid. To create this naturally at home, mix 1 tablespoon of white vinegar (which contains acetic acid) into 1 cup of willow bark tea.

377 Salicylate herbs include: Black haw (*Viburnum prunifolium*), cramp bark (*Viburnum opulus*), marshmallow root (*althaea officinalis*), meadowsweet (*Filipendula ulmaria)*, sweet birch (*Betula lenta*), white birch (*Betula papyrifera*) white willow bark (*salix alba*), and wintergreen (*Gaultheria procumbens*). This is not a comprehensive list, consult with a competent herbalist.

risk for kidney stones. May interact with laxatives, blood thinners, or digoxin medications.

YLANG YLANG:
Cananga odorata

Clinical studies have shown that, not only can the aroma of the essential oil of ylang ylang lower blood pressure, heart rate, depression and nervousness,[378] but applying it topically to the skin also provides the same positive effects.[379] When used topically it must be combined with a carrier oil (vegetable or mineral oil) at the ratio of 12 drops of ylang ylang oil to 2 tablespoons (60ml) of carrier oil. Ylang ylang blends well with bergamot oil if you want to create a therapeutic anti-anxiety blend. *Precautions: Never use essentials oils at full strength on the skin to reduce the risk of sensitization.*

ZINC:

Zinc is an essential mineral in our diets necessary for the formation of white blood cells and helps synthesize the proteins our cells need for healthy growth. The recommended daily intake for zinc is 11mg for adult men and 8mg for adult women. Do not consumer more than a daily intake of 40mg (counting for diet, medicinal, and supplemental intake) unless your doctor recommends otherwise. Dietary sources of zinc include oysters (which are very high in zinc), beef, lamb, crab, lobster, wheat germ, nuts, fortified cereals, pumpkin seeds and squash seeds. If you take a zinc supplement you should know that phytochemicals in legumes and whole grains may hinder absorption of zinc, so do not take your supplement with a meal. If taking it with water is too hard on your stomach take it with milk instead. Chemotherapy may reduce zinc levels in your body, which in turn may cause you lose your sense of taste to a degree. If this happens then I recommend that you discuss with your doctor whether you need a zinc supplement. Be cautious though; there is some evidence that zinc may interfere with platinum-based chemotherapy medications when taken above the daily recommended amounts. Be sure to discuss this with your oncologist if you have concerns. *Precautions: Too much zinc can be harmful, do not take more than the recommended amount given by your physician. Zinc may decrease the effectiveness of certain antibiotics. It may increase the side effects of the chemotherapy drug cisplatin. Very large doses of zinc can cause copper and iron deficiencies as well as be toxic. Diuretic medications may decrease your systemic zinc levels; speak to your doctor if you are concerned.*

---

378 *Effects of Ylang-Ylang aroma on blood pressure and heart rate in healthy men.* (Jung, 2013)
379 *Relaxing Effect of Ylang Ylang Oil on Humans After Transdermal Absorption.*
    (Hongratanaworkakit, 2006).

Chapter 7
CYP3A4 ENZYMES and CHEMOTHERAPY

CYP3A4[380] is an important enzyme found in your liver and intestinal tract. This enzyme is necessary for the metabolism of certain medications and substances. Medications and substances which rely on CYP3A4 for metabolization are known as "CYP3A4 substrates" (hereafter referred to as "substrates"). Certain medications, herbs, and foods affect the action of this enzyme which, in turn, affects the action of the substrates consumed. Because several chemotherapy agents are substrates of this enzyme this chapter takes a look at what this means and how it affects your prescribed treatment plan.

CYP3A4 INDUCERS
Certain medications, herbs, and foods are known as CYP3A4 inducers, which means these items *increase* the action of the enzyme. This increase in action results in the accelerated metabolism and elimination of the substrate. This accelerated process causes the substrate to be removed too quickly from your body resulting in having too-little time to perform its therapeutic action. If the substrate happens to be your chemotherapy agent this would mean your agent will not have enough time to deliver its full effect against your cancer. This may require a dose increase which increases the risk of side effects. Some of the most commonly known natural CYP3A4 inducers include: DHEA,[381] echinacea, garlic, ginkgo biloba, nicotine-containing products, St. John's wort, foods containing tangeretin,[382] and valerian root. Consuming any of these during treatment with chemotherapy substrates runs the risk of metabolizing the agent too quickly for your benefit. Chemotherapy-based substrates affected by inducers include the following:

Afatinib	Axitinib	Bortezomib
Bosutinib	Cabazitaxel	Cabozantinib
Ceritinib	Cobimetinib	Crizotinib
Dabrafenib	Dasatinib	Enzalutammide
Erlotinib	Everolimus	Exemestane
Ibrutinib	Idelalisib	Ifosfamide
Imatinib	Irinotecan	Ixabepilone
Ixazomib	Lapatinib	Nilotinib

---

380 The full name for CYP 34A = Cytochrome P450-34A . Although there are also other CYP enzymes, for the sake of simplicity, I will focus only on CYP3A4 in this chapter.
381 Also known as dehydroepiandrosterone
382 Tangeretin is a bitter tasting flavonoid present in the peels of most citrus fruits , a.k.a. the "zest". This substance can also be found as a natural supplement.

Olaparib	Osimertinib	Palbociclib
Panobinostat	Ponatinib Hydrochloride	Prednisone
Regorafenib	Romidepsin	Sonidegib
Sorafenib Tosylate	Sunitinib Malate	Temsirolimus
Toremifene	Trabectedin	Vandetanib
Venetoclax	Vincristine Lipid Complex	Vincristine Sulfate
Vincristine Sulfate Liposome		

** Take note that sometimes a single medication may contain some ingredients which are inducers and some which are inhibitors. Because the above table is not a comprehensive list I advise you to speak with your prescribing physicians.

A number of other pharmaceuticals, both prescription and over-the-counter, are also known to be inducers meaning these will also accelerate the metabolism of the above-listed substrates. To view a listing of pharmaceutical inducers to avoid when taking the above-listed substrates please see Appendix 1 of this book. Please note: If your medication is on the list in appendix 1 do not suddenly stop taking it without consulting with your prescribing doctor first. If you find that you are on a medication that will affect your chemotherapy agent you have two choices: (a) Your oncologist may be able to prescribe a different chemotherapy agent for you, or (b) Your prescribing doctor(s) may be able to prescribe a different medication that will work with your chemotherapy agent(s).

If you are on any of the above-listed chemotherapy agents do not consume any CYP3A4 inducers for two weeks prior to use of the affected agent, during use of the agent, and for at least two weeks after you are finished using the agent. Speak to your prescribing physicians if this requires you to change your medications.

CYP3A4 INHIBITORS

The CYP3A4 inhibitors work the opposite way from inducers; instead of inducing the enzyme to metabolize the substrates too fast, these actually *inhibit* the metabolization of the substrates causing the processing and elimination to be *too slow*. This means that the drugs will hang around in your system much longer than they are intended for. Though this may seem like a good thing initially, in reality it is not. Allow me to illustrate:

Let's say a patient is prescribed a substrate, Plendil, for his high blood pressure. The patient is instructed to take only one tablet per day; this means it takes a normal, healthy body 24 hours to process the drug properly out of the system through the CYP3A4 "pathway" before the next dose is due. If, however, this patient is in the habit of drinking a glass of grapefruit juice – a known inhibitor – with his breakfast every day he is slowing down the metabolization of the drug. As a result, when he takes the next dose with more grapefruit juice he has more Plendil in his system than he is supposed to because the previous dose has not been fully metabolized due to juice's enzyme inhibition.[383] If this continues for several days his system will quickly become congested with excess Plendil trying to be processed through a bottle-necked pathway. This will quickly build up toxic levels of the drug in his system causing side effects and possibly other health issues. And, since a single glass of grapefruit juice has been shown to inhibit the metabolization of drugs for up to three days in some cases,[384] you can see where this quickly becomes a problem. Imagine if this were your chemotherapy agent instead.

Many foods and supplements are CYP3A4 inhibitors, such as: Agaricus sylvaticus/A. blazei mushrooms, American ginseng (*Panax quinquefolius*), angelica (*Angelica dahurica*), Asian ginseng (*Panax ginseng*), astragalus (*Astragalus membranaceus*), barberry (*berberis*), berberine, black cohosh (*Actaea racemosa*), black cumin,[385] black pepper (*piper nigrum*),[386] bergamot (*Citrus bergamia*), blood oranges (a.k.a. Seville orange),[387] boswellia (*Boswellia serrata*), broccoli, bromelain, carambola/star fruit,[388] cat's claw (*Uncaria tomentosa*), cauliflower, cloves,[389] cranberry products, coptis (*Coptis chinensis*),, devil's claw (*Harpagophytum procumbens*), dragon fruit, echinacea (*Echinacea purpurea/E. angustifolia*), garlic,[390] ginkgo (*Ginkgo biloba*), goldenseal (*Hydrastis canadensis*),[391] grapefruit,[392] grape products (red/purple),[393] grape seed extract, guava products, khella (*Ammi visnaga*),[394] kiwi/Chinese gooseberry, licorice root (*Glycyrrhiza glabra*), mango, naringenin compounds;[395] neem (*Azadirachta indica*),[396] Oregon grape (*Mahonia aquifolium*), papaya, passion fruit, pawpaw,[397] pineapple, piperine,[398] pomegranate, pomelo, quercetin,raisins (dark), rambutan, red wine,[399] reishi

---

383According to one study a single glass of grapefruit juice significantly augmented the affects of Plendil *"Management of Grapefruit-Drug Interactions"* (Stump, 2006)

384*Relationship between time after intake of grapefruit juice and the effect on pharmacokinetics and pharmacodynamics of nisoldipine in healthy subjects* (Takanaga, 2000)

385Some studies have shown black cumin seed to have a 41% inhibition rate.

386Black pepper contains piperine, which some studies have shown an 84% inhibition rate at doses of 20 mg. Black pepper contains roughly 7% piperine. A single 1/8 tsp. serving of black pepper will contain roughly 40mg of piperine.

387 Blood oranges/Seville oranges are often used in the manufacture of marmalade.

388 T he inhibition of star fruit was stronger than that of grapefruit.

389 The eugenol in cloves is a potent inhibitor. Topically used clove oil is much safer.

390Garlic is known as both an inhibitor and an inducer. One property doesn't necessarily cancel out the other. It is safer to just avoid it altogether when using drugs which are affects by CYP3A4)

391Some studies have shown goldenseal to have a 40% inhibition rate.

392Some studies have shown a single serving of grapefruit product to have a 62% inhibition rate. The fruit, the juice, and supplemental extracts are all CYP3A4 inhibitors. Flavonoids in grapefruit which contribute to this include bergapten, naringenin, naringin, and quercetin.

393Red and purple grapes contain resveratrol, which is a CYP3A4 inhibitor. Green grapes do not contain resveratrol.

394Also known as toothpick weed, toothpick plant, and bisnaga.

395Found in items such as grapefruit, oranges, and cooked tomato products.

396Also known as Nimtree and Indian Lilac.

397Although papaya and paw paws are in the same species (*carica papaya*), these are distinctly different fruits. Paw paw is not the same as American paw paw.

398Derived from black pepper. Some studies have shown piperine to have an 84% inhibition rate at doses of 20mg.

399Red wine contains resveratrol, a known CYP3A4 inhibitor. White wine does not contain resveratrol.

(*Ganoderma lucidum*), resveratrol, sea badara (*Strychnos Ligustrina, a.k.a. Strychnos Lucida*), [400] tangerines, tree turmeric (*Berberis aristata*), and Valencia oranges. Just as with the Plendil example mentioned earlier, if you consume any of these items while taking a substrate chemo agent you will increase your chance of developing worsening side effects and possible organ damage, depending upon the chemo agent involved. Chemotherapy drugs which can become toxic when used with CYP3A4 inhibitors include (listed by generic names):

Ado-trastuzumab Emtansine	Axitinib	Bexarotene
Bortezomib	Bosutinib	Cabazitaxel
Cabozantinib	Ceritinib	Cobimetinib
Crizotinib	Dasatinib	Erlotinib
Ibrutinib	Idelalisib	Ifosfamide
Imatinib	Irinotecan Hydrochloride	Ixabepilone
Lapatinib Ditosylate	Nanoparticle Paclitaxel	Nilotinib
Olaparib	Paclitaxel	Palbociclib
Panobinostat	Pazopanib Hydrochloride	Ponatinib Hydrochloride
Prednisone	Regorafenib	Romidepsin
Ruxolitinib Phosphate	Sonidegib	Sunitinib Malate
Temsirolimus	Toremifene	Trabectedin
Venetoclax		

** Take note that sometimes a single medication may contain some ingredients which are inducers and some which are inhibitors. Because the above table is not a comprehensive list I advise you to speak with your prescribing physicians.

If you are on any of the above-listed chemotherapy agents, do not consume CYP3A4 inhibitors for two weeks prior to use of the agent, during use of the agent, and for at least two weeks after you are finished using the agent. To view a list of pharmaceutical inhibitors to avoid, please see Appendix 2 of this book. Please note: If your medication is on the list in appendix 2 do not suddenly stop taking it without consulting with your prescribing doctor first. If you find that you are on a medication that will affect your chemotherapy agent you have two choices: (a) Your oncologist may be able to prescribe a different chemotherapy agent for you, or (b) Your other prescribing doctors may be able to prescribe a different medication that will work with your chemotherapy agent(s).

Is it really *that* important to be careful about using inducers and inhibitors with certain medication? YES. Let me illustrate this importance by using the

---

400Also known as Bidara Laut and Wood Snake.

chemotherapy agent imatinib as an example, since it is sensitive to both inducers and inhibitors:

St. John's wort – an inducer – is a commonly used supplement taken for depression, insomnia, and stomach upset. This herb can be useful in many cases, however, for a patient on imatinib to treat leukemia St. John's wort can reduce the patient's levels of imatinib by a significant 30%. This means that nearly one third of the treatment is being wasted because it is rendered less effective by hurried metabolism! This requires increasing the dose of imatinib, thus increasing the risk of developing side effects and possibly other health problems.

Inhibitors are no better. Licorice root contains glabidin, a substance which has been shown in some studies to have a 70% inhibition rate. This means that a patient who is prescribed imatinib who is using licorice root will have a large amount of the previous dose of imatinib leftover in his system when taking the next dose. This means he will have the new full dose, plus a large amount of the previous dose concurrent in his system, effectively causing too much to be in the system. If this patient continues to use the licorice root this continual "congestion" of imatinib building up will greatly increase the side effects of the imatinib causing the patient great discomfort and distress. If left unchecked this can even cause the imatinib to build up to toxic levels which can permanently damage the liver. This requires decreasing the dose of imatinib in order to reduce the risks of toxicity; and a reduction in dose *may* give your cancer the upper hand.

Clearly, knowing which chemotherapy agents are CYP3A4 substrates is very important when it comes to effective chemotherapy management. If you find that your particular combination of chemotherapy agents makes it difficult to figure out which foods and supplements to accept or avoid do not hesitate to consult with a competent, experienced practitioner to help you.

Please keep aware that medical science is constantly creating newer medications and chemotherapy agents on a regular basis, therefore the lists in this chapter and the referenced appendices may not be complete. If you are on a medication or chemotherapy agent which is not mentioned in these lists do not hesitate to ask your prescribing physicians if you are taking anything that is affected by the CYP3A4 enzyme.

Chapter 8
HOLISTIC DIETARY GUIDELINES

INTRODUCTION

Many patients looking for additional ways to beat their cancers often consider following "cancer diets" which are supposed to be designed to help their bodies fight the cancer and cope with the stresses of treatment. When looking at these diet regimens you must be sure to consider the following first:

- Do you have any special needs in your diet? This would include food allergies, food sensitivities, diabetes, bowel disorders, low cholesterol diets, low sodium diets, fluid restrictions, dialysis diets, vegan/vegetarian diets, etc. Be sure the "cancer diet" you are interested in accommodates your dietary needs.

- Make sure the diet is scientifically based and balanced. Do not hesitate to consult with a properly educated nutritionist or a registered dietitian to confirm the balance of the diet.

- Be sure no elements of the diet will cause interactions or adverse effects with your medications or chemotherapy. For example, if a diet requires frequent consumption of grapefruit then you must first make sure your current treatment regimen does not include medications or agents which interact with grapefruit.

- Be sure to consult with your physician first before making any sudden changes to your diet. Not only does he or she need to know what you are doing so that treatments can be adjusted if necessary, but your doctor may also have other insights for your dietary needs that you should know.

ANTIOXIDANTS

There is a lot of conflicting information as to whether a cancer patient should take antioxidant supplements during a course of chemotherapy treatment. Before getting into the discussion about this let me first explain what antioxidants are and what they do for your body:

Simply put, an antioxidant is a substance which prevents damage to body cells caused by oxidation. Oxidation is a process in which atoms lose some of their electrons, and it has everything to do with oxygen and how it is used: Within your body cells oxygen is a key element necessary for generating energy from the various nutrients that we consume such as sugar, fatty acids and amino acids. This is done by removing electrons from the molecules of the nutrients and adding them to other molecules and atoms, including oxygen. When this happens, the molecules that are missing their electrons become unstable "free radicals" which take the needed electrons from stable molecules located nearby in order to re-stabilize. When these stable molecules are "robbed" of their electrons, they in turn become free radicals which then steal from the stable molecules located near *them*, thus perpetuating the cycle. Although these free radicals are a normal part of metabolism, sometimes these can be created in excess in response to pollution, tobacco exposure, radiation, and chemical exposure (including food additives and preservatives). This excess of free radicals can be very disruptive to the affected cells resulting in problems that may eventually lead to the mutations which start cancer. This is where antioxidants come in to play: Antioxidants come around and donate *their own* electrons to the de-stabilized atoms; this stabilizes the atoms so they do not continue a cycle of electron "robbery" with other atoms, thereby resolving the situation. Because antioxidants remain stable even *after* donating their atoms, the oxidation process is brought to a grinding halt and cell damage (and the risk of cancer) is greatly reduced. This protective action is why consuming antioxidants is such an important part of a healthy diet.[401]

Now, this is where it can become confusing to patients: Because some types of chemotherapy agents kill cancer by *generating* free radicals (thus damaging the cancer cells) it would be contrary to use excessive antioxidants with those types of agents. In some circles it is thought that, although antioxidants protect healthy cells from becoming damaged, the antioxidants may also help protect cancerous cells from the damaging effects of chemotherapy and radiation treatments. In other circles it is believed that, since you do not want more of your healthy cells becoming damaged and risking further cancer, you should continue taking antioxidants as a protective measure against the chemotherapy – especially since cancer patients tend to have low levels of antioxidants in their systems to begin with. This becomes even more confusing if you start looking into the scientific studies because some have found evidence to support the use of antioxidants while other studies remain inconclusive. There are even some which suggest that only particular antioxidants should be avoided. With such opposing views it is easy to see why a cancer patient would become confused about his or her intake of antioxidants.

The biggest problem here is that there are so many variables among cancer patients and chemotherapy agents that it is impossible to make a blanket statement on the matter. Variables such as the types of cancers, the patient's genetics, the stages of the cancers, the treatments and holistic therapies being used by the patients, ages of the patients, risk factors the patients were exposed to, the general health of the patients, etc. all make a difference in the outcome of each individual. So then, how can you decide what you should do in regard to antioxidant supplementation?

First, speak with your oncologist to see if your cancer treatment regimen involves using free radicals to destroy your cancer. If so, then you need to avoid antioxidant *supplementation* unless your oncologist recommends otherwise. You also need to let your qualified herbalist know about these treatments because some products, such as grape seed or pine bark, contain strong antioxidants in them. Unless your oncologist states otherwise, normal dietary sources of antioxidants[402] in normal amounts should be safe to consume during treatment.

If you are *not* on a free radical-based chemotherapy regimen be sure you take

---

401 Some nutrients which are known to be antioxidant include: Vitamins C and E, carotenoids, lycopene, glutathione, flavonoids, polyphenols, alpha-lipoic acids (ALA), and ubiquinol.

402 Dietary sources of antioxidants include, but are not limited to: All berries, natural process dark chocolate, grapes, nuts, and dark green leafy vegetables.

the recommendations from your oncologist, qualified herbalist, registered dietitian, or nutritionist. Educate yourself on interactions between antioxidant supplements and medications you are currently taking, and be sure to keep all things in moderation. If your health care team decides an antioxidant supplement is good for your situation then take only the recommended amount as some antioxidants can actually become toxic if taken in excess.

SACCHARINE

Artificial sweeteners are chemically made sweeteners used in place of natural sugars such as alcohol sugars, cane sugar, beet sugar, and honey. Artificial sweeteners tend to be popular because they are cheaper to produce than natural sweeteners and they are much lower in calories and carbohydrates. Aside from the irony that artificial sweeteners tend to promote obesity[403] it is widely thought that these sweeteners also promote the development of cancer and other health issues. What is the truth in this matter?

The laboratory tests which linked artificial sweeteners to cancer used enormous quantities of the sweeteners, far beyond what a normal diet could possibly have. This is no different than using excessive quantities of vitamin A, vitamin D, or Iron – all of which are extremely toxic when taken in excessive amounts. The one artificial sweetener in particular that got a bad reputation is one known as saccharine: commercially known by names such as "Sweet-n-low" and "Sweet Twin." Several decades ago researchers observed a link between saccharine and the development of cancer in laboratory rats and this prompted a law requiring a warning on food products which contained the sweetener. However, in the 1990's further research found that the mechanism which led to cancer in rats was irrelevant in humans as the chemical process metabolizes very differently in the human body. As a result, the FDA no longer required the food label warning, and in 2010 the Environmental Protection Agency released the statement that it was deleting saccharine from its list of carcinogens. In March of 2015 the American Chemical Society released information showing that saccharine can actually be used as an agent to *fight* cancer. At the 249th National Meeting and Exposition of the American Chemical Society, Dr. Robert McKenna, Ph. D. of the University of Florida[404] presented findings that saccharin blocks a protein known as carbonic anhydrase IX (a.k.a. "CA9"), a protein which encourages the growth of aggressive cancers in organs such as the lungs, liver, kidneys, pancreas, brain, and breasts.[405] This protein is not typically found in healthy human cells, therefore saccharine has the potential to be developed as a targeted therapy treatment for certain cancers. Research is currently investigating this matter.

NATURAL SWEETENERS/CARBOHYDRATES

Natural sweeteners include products such as alcohol sugars, cane sugar, beet

---

403 *Fueling the Obesity Epidemic? Artificially Sweetened Beverage Use and Long-term Weight Gain.* (Fowler, 2008)
404 Dr. McKenna is a professor in the Dept of Biochemistry and Molecular Biology at the university.
405 These findings were based on early research performed by Dr. Claudius T. Supuran, Ph. D Of the University of Florence, Italy, and Dr. Sally-Ann Poulsen, Ph. D Of Griffith University in Australia.

sugar, honey, real maple syrup, pure stevia, fruit sugars, and molasses. Carbohydrates are starches and other substances which are broken down into sugars by your body. Sources of carbohydrates include grains, milk, root vegetables, peas, bananas, plantains, taro, and winter squash. When you consume natural sugars and other carbohydrates your body converts them to glucose, an energy source used by every cell in your body. Unfortunately, cancer cells tend to *especially* prefer glucose and use it as their primary fuel source (see chapter 2 of this book, subheading "*Cachexia*" for more details). This fact leads many to believe that consuming natural sugars and other carbohydrates will actually feed their cancers; ergo they eliminate all of these from their diet. What is the truth to this belief?

To begin with, no large clinical studies have observed sugar or carbohydrates accelerating the growth of cancer and no large clinical studies have observed that the elimination of these food items stops or slows cancer growth. In reality, if you completely eliminate these items from your diet your body will still require glucose for its *healthy* cells and will thus break down muscle tissue in order to obtain the glucose it needs. In essence, you are starving your healthy cells, weakening your body *and* running a high risk of malnutrition by following such a stripped down diet.

Does this mean you can eat all the sugar and carbohydrates you want? No. Excessive consumption of sugars and carbohydrates will cause a high increase in your blood's insulin levels. Insulin is a hormone which is released to help your body use the glucose made from the foods you eat, ergo the more glucose there is in your system the more insulin your body releases in order to take care of it. This is where it gets interesting: Insulin encourages cancer to grow; in fact insulin is the substance researchers use to grow cancer cells in their labs for research. Therefore, what you need to do is consume enough sugar/carbohydrates to keep your healthy cells happy while at the same time ensuring you are not causing excessive releases of insulin in your body.[406] Generally speaking, "enough" sugars/carbohydrates usually means up to 5 servings of fruits and vegetables, 3 servings of dairy, and 6 servings of grain daily. Stay away from all sweet treats and snacks, and trade out your high carb snacks for lower-carb alternatives. To prevent insulin "spikes" (sudden increases) you should eat whole grains instead of processed grains and have some protein with your sugar/carbs, as these habits will help slow the glucose conversion thus reducing the risk of insulin spikes. Consult with a competent nutritionist or registered dietitian to be sure you are correctly balancing your diet. Some patients choose to exchange their regular cane sugar for alcohol sugars.[407] An alcohol sugar, which looks like regular cane sugar, is a natural sugar derived from certain plants. Because these sugars have a lower level of carbohydrates in them they are safer for cancer patients to consume. You can identify alcohol sugars by the suffix "-*itol*" in their names (sorbitol, xylitol, erythritol, etc.). Alcohol sugars do not contain ethanol, therefore they can be safely used by recovering alcoholics. What's more, two particular alcohol sugars have been shown to help hinder cancer growth:

---

406 If you are a diabetic patient using insulin products speak with your prescribing physician regarding your dosage levels. Never stop taking your prescribed insulin without your physician's advice.
407 Alcohol sugars may cause a laxative effect in some people. Therefore take caution if you are already experiencing diarrhea as a side effect of your chemotherapy treatments.

117

Sorbitol: Some in vitro laboratory tests have shown sorbitol to cause cell death in cancer cells.[408] However, it must also be noted that another study found that heat-shock pre-treatment of certain cancers may protect them from the effects of sorbitol.[409] Therefore, if you are a cancer patient using any kind of heat therapy and you are interested in using sorbitol I strongly advise you to speak with your practitioner and/or physician who is performing your heat therapy regimen first.

Xylitol: This is an alcohol sugar found in some chewing gums as well as in bulk packages in some natural food stores. This sweetener has a known anti-inflammatory effect making it attractive as a sweetener for cancer patients, especially for those at risk for cachexia. What's more, in vitro testing has shown xylitol to inhibit the growth of certain lung cancers. [410]

INFLAMMATION DIET

Inflammation is a normal physical reaction to foreign invaders in the body. It happens when your immune system detects that invaders have entered the body (virus, bacteria, fungus, mold, protozoa, amoebae, etc.) and quickly acts to destroy the invaders before they multiply and cause bodily harm. In most cases this process of inflammation is a *good* thing that protects us from certain illness. However, in some cases chronic inflammation can be caused by factors other than microscopic invaders; oftentimes it is caused by a diet consistently filled with a high concentration of the following:

- ***Saturated fats***: Any *natural* fat that is not liquid at normal room temperature (68 °F or 20 °C) is a saturated fat. This includes red meats, coconut oil, cheese, lard, and palm oil. Also, any dairy item made from any milk (except for skim) also contains saturated fats, such as sour cream, heavy cream, light cream, butter, ice cream, and anything made with these ingredients.

- ***Trans fats***: These are liquid fats which are made solid through a process of hydrogenation (i.e. adding hydrogen to the fat). Although this includes both fully hydrogenated fats *and* partially hydrogenated fats, some companies consider only fully hydrogenated oils to be a trans fat. Therefore, when you read your food labels be sure that they do not include any kind of hydrogenated fats. Trans fats are found nearly everywhere in the commercial world such as shortening, pastries, some peanut butters, fried foods, margarine, commercial snacks, coffee creamers, and many other sources. Because trans fats are so unhealthy the FDA has required commercial food companies to cease using trans fats in their products by 2018. However, this does not mean that all other countries in the world will follow suit, so be sure to check your labels when consuming foods made in other countries.

- ***Omega fatty acids***: It seems that we always hear about the anti-inflammatory health benefits of using omega 3 fatty acids, but we do not hear so much about

408*Sorbitol induces apoptosis of human colorectal cancer cells via p38 MAPK signal transduction* (Xue Lu, 2014)

409*Heat-shock pretreatment inhibits sorbitol-induced apoptosis in K562, U937 and HeLa cells* (Gabriella Marfe, 2009)

410*Xylitol induces cell death in lung cancer A549 cells by autophagy.* (Park, 2015)

the omega 6 fatty acids or omega 9 fatty acids.[411] Although all three types of fatty acids are important for our nutritional needs, omega 6's tend to cause inflammation when taken without enough omega 3's to tame them. Therefore you want to avoid food items which contain high levels of omega 6's, such as: Corn oil, cottonseed oil, soybean oil, and sunflower oil. You need to try for an Omega 6/Omega 3 ratio of 2:1, or as close to that as possible. Since the average diet in the United States tends to have a ratio of about 20:1, or ten times the recommended amount of omega 6's, this may require serious dietary changes. Due to the large amount of fat-containing foods available it can seem a little tricky to figure out what you should and should not be consuming. Therefore the following table is provided to help you see at a glance the percentages of fats and fatty acids in common cooking fats:

Fat	Saturated *percentage*	Omega 3 *percentage*	Omega 6 *percentage*	Omega 9 *percentage*
Almond oil	8.00%	0.00%	17.00%	69.00%
Avocado oil	11.00%	1.00%	12.50%	67.00%
Butterfat	68.00%	1.00%	3.00%	28.00%
Canola oil	7.00%	11.00%	21.00%	61.00%
Coconut oil	91.00%	0.00%	2.00%	7.00%
Corn oil	13.00%	1.00%	57.00%	29.00%
Cottonseed oil	27.00%	Trace	54.00%	19.00%
Flax seed oil	9.00%	57.00%	18.00%	16.00%
Grape seed oil	10.00%	0.10%	70.00%	16.00%
Lard	43.00%	1.00%	9.00%	47.00%
Olive oil	15.00%	1.00%	9.00%	75.00%
Palm oil	51.00%	Trace	10.00%	39.00%
Peanut oil	19.00%	Trace	33.00%	48.00%
Safflower oil	8.00%	1.00%	14.00%	77.00%
Sesame oil	14.00%	0.30%	41.00%	39.00%
Soybean oil	15.00%	8.00%	54.00%	23.00%
Sunflower oil	12.00%	1.00%	71.00%	16.00%

411 Although omega 3's and omega 6's are known as "essential" (we MUST get them from our diets), omega 9's are non-essential, which means our bodies can produce this fatty acids when needed. Therefore the amounts of omega 9's in a food item is not a requirement when choosing your fats. Omega 6 fatty acids support our immune system and omega 9 fatty acids help protect our arteries from plaque buildup.

Fat	Saturated *percentage*	Omega 3 *percentage*	Omega 6 *percentage*	Omega 9 *percentage*
Walnut oil	9.00%	10.00%	52.00%	22.00%

- ***Refined sugars and carbohydrates***: Refined sugars and carbohydrates come from over-processed sugars and grains such as white sugar, high fructose corn syrup, white flour, white rice, ramen noodles, de-germed cornmeal, white pasta and many cold breakfast cereals. Because these are refined they break down in your digestive system more quickly resulting in a stronger sugar rush into your system. This over-abundance of sugar overwhelms your system which tries to cope by signaling your pancreas to produce large amounts of insulin (a hormone required for properly metabolizing sugar). Because your body is designed to handle smaller amounts of insulin at a time, this flood of insulin causes system-wide inflammation. Using *unrefined* sugars and grains, however, break down much slower in your system, allowing your body to keep up with the pace of sugar being released. Therefore, instead of using refined sugars and grains it is better to use natural, unrefined products such as raw honey, molasses, real maple syrup, whole grains, brown rice, quinoa, millet and bran cereals. Please keep in mind that using unrefined sources is not a license to eat large amounts of them. Keep your diet balanced, especially if you are diabetic.

- ***Gluten***: Gluten is a protein present in certain grains such as wheat,[412] rye, barley, triticale,[413] brewer's yeast, seitan, wheat starch, vital wheat gluten, and malt. People sensitive to gluten should eat gluten free grains such as: Brown rice, corn, oats, amaranth, buckwheat, millet, quinoa, hato mugi, teff, and wild rice. Always read your food labels, as some items that look to be gluten free may actually have gluten-based ingredients in them such as malt, flour, or dextrin. Be aware that gluten-based ingredients may also show up in surprising ways. For example, gluten-free french fries may be cooked in oil that is shared with batter-coated onion rings. Please note that gluten is only inflammatory in people who are sensitive to this protein, therefore, if you do *not* have gluten sensitivities then you do not need to worry about your gluten intake. If you are unsure whether you have gluten sensitivities I strongly advise you to speak with your doctor and be assessed.

- ***Dairy***: "Dairy" includes any food that is primarily milk based. This can include milk from any mammal such as buffalo, camels, cows, goats, sheep, etc. Some people are unable to properly digest milk sugar, known as lactose. Such ones are known as lactose intolerant and this causes severe digestive issues such as diarrhea, stomach cramps, and excessive gas. Other people are allergic to milk based proteins such as whey or casein. This may cause the same symptoms as lactose intolerance but may also include severe symptoms

---

412 Wheat products include ingredients such as: Durum, semolina, wheat berries, emmer, spelt, farina, farro, graham, kamut, and einkorn.

413 Triticale is a hybrid grain crossed from rye and wheat.

such as rash, hives, or difficulties with breathing. People who are lactose intolerant or who have an allergy to dairy will experience inflammation when they consume products containing dairy-based ingredients.[414] If you are neither lactose intolerant nor allergic to dairy then dairy products should not cause inflammation in your system.

KETOGENIC DIET

A ketogenic diet is a diet which focuses on burning calories from fats and proteins instead of from carbohydrates. This is called a ketogenic diet because the metabolic process for burning fats and proteins for energy results in the production of ketones; an energy source alternative to the glucose energy produced through carbohydrates. A typical ketogenic regimen usually contains about 75% healthy fats, 20% proteins, and a meager 5% of carbohydrates.

Oftentimes cancer patients are advised by their holistic practitioners to follow a ketogenic diet because cancer cells tend to prefer glucose as their primary source of energy. The idea is that, if you take away the glucose (via eliminating most carbohydrates), you starve the cancer cells and slow the growth of tumors. Does this dietary regimen actually work?

As of this writing there are numerous clinical trials on human patients studying the effects of a ketogenic diet in cancer patients, however information at this time is scant. One pilot study using 16 patients with advanced metastatic tumors was conducted. Out of the 16 patients only 6 completed the study, reporting *"improved emotional functioning and less insomnia."* [415] One report on two pediatric cancer cases showed one patient experienced *"significant clinical improvements in mood"* and continued the diet for a year *"remaining free of disease progression."* [416] Another case study showed a 65 year old patient using a ketogenic diet along with conventional therapy showed no evidence of her brain tumor after two months on a ketogenic diet; ten weeks after ceasing the diet MRI evidence of the tumor recurrence began to show.[417] Although these cases are encouraging, keep in mind that the numbers of patients is very small, therefore it is not yet known if these are typical responses or simply individual responses.

If you choose to use a ketogenic diet there are many precautions you must take as this type of diet is very stressful for the body and can cause more harm than good if not done under competent, professional supervision. For example, if you begin to consume an excessive amount of protein you may damage your kidneys. Or, if you consume too many of the wrong kinds of fats you can cause serious cholesterol and heart problems. A person using a ketogenic diet is also at risk for certain nutritional

---

414Dairy based ingredients include: Casein, caseinates, anything with the word "butter", hydrolysates, lactoglobulin, lactalbumin, lactose, cream ghee, whey, lactoferrin, nougat, paneer, and cream.

415*Effects of a Ketogenic Diet on the Quality of Life in 16 Patient with Advanced Cancer: A Pilot Trial* (Schmidt, 2011)

416*Effects of a Ketogenic Diet on Tumor Metabolism and Nutritional Status in Pediatric Oncology Patients: Two Case Reports* (Nebeling, 1995)

417*Metabolic Management of Glioblastoma Multiforme Using Standard Therapy Together with a Restricted Ketogenic Diet: Case Report*: (Zuccoli, 2010)

deficiencies. I strongly recommend that you seek professional guidance if you choose to follow a ketogenic diet.

Ketogenic dieting is not for everyone. Some pre-existing health conditions can make such a diet extremely harmful, even deadly, for some patients. If you have any of the following conditions be sure your physicians and practitioners know before using a ketogenic diet:

- Fat metabolism disorders
- Gastric bypass surgery
- History of pancreatitis
- Hormonal disorders
- Gall bladder disease
- Metabolic disorders
- Abdominal tumors
- Pregnant/lactating
- Sluggish bowels
- Kidney disease
- Epilepsy (adult)
- Liver disease
- Diabetes

RAW FOOD DIET

Many people promote a raw food diet for maximum health. A raw food diet is a system of eating in which no food is heated past 118°F (47.7 °C) The main theory behind this diet is that, since Adam and Eve likely lived on a raw food diet and did well, then today it should still be the best diet for us. Proponents of raw food diets teach that raw foods contain more enzymes and nutrients than cooked foods and are therefore better for one's health and well-being. This diet not only includes raw fruits, vegetables, and nuts, but may also include the consumption of raw and unpasteurized milk, eggs, meats, and fish if the consumer is not following a vegan diet.

Let's talk about the raw plant foods first: Although it is true that most fruits, vegetables, and nuts are better for you when eaten raw it is also true that there are definite exceptions to this rule. For example freshly harvested cashew nuts are naturally covered in a toxic layer that must be roasted in order to deactivate the toxins for safe consumption.[418] Some vegetables, especially in the cabbage family,[419] contain substances called goitrogens which can block essential thyroid hormones and therefore must be lightly cooked to deactivate the goitrogens. Other vegetables[420]

---

418 "Raw" cashews are put through this single roasting process. "Roasted" cashews are put through a second roasting process.

419 The cabbage family vegetables are also known as cruciferous vegetables. These include all kinds of cabbages, arugula, kale, turnips, rutabagas, collard greens, Brussels sprouts, broccoli, radishes, watercress, mustard greens, Kohlrabi, and broccoli.

420 These types of vegetables include asparagus, carrots, kale, mushrooms, peppers, pumpkin, and tomatoes

have tougher cell walls which lock in the essential nutrients and thus require light cooking in order to soften the cell walls enough to release the full load of nutrients. Other raw foods, such as spinach or purslane, contain high amounts of oxalic acid, a substance which prevents the absorption of certain nutrients and may contribute to the formation of kidney stones. Fortunately, oxalic acid is easily leached out by water, therefore it is better to blanch these types of vegetables rather than eating them raw (Blanching = placing the food in boiling water for three minutes, then remove). When lightly cooking be careful you do not overcook so that you leave as many nutrients intact as possible. "Lightly cooked" means 45 seconds in the microwave, or 2 minutes steamed, or 3 minutes sauteed. I only recommend boiling for the removal of oxalic acid; I do not recommend boiling otherwise because this method tends to also leach other nutrients out into the cooking water. If boiling is the only heating method available to you then do not boil for longer than 2-3 minutes. It is also important to be aware that foods containing vitamins A, D, E, and K require a small amount of heart-healthy fats to go with them in order to absorb those vitamins fully in your system.

As for raw animal products, there are other health issues to be aware of. It is well documented that raw dairy, meats, and fish can carry salmonella, E. coli, hepatitis,and parasites. All of these diseases can cause extreme illness and death even in healthy people A patient with cancer, especially one undergoing therapies that may lower his or her immune system, is much more susceptible to contracting these raw-food diseases. Cooking these items will not ruin the nutrition in them and will save you the trouble of a terrible illness or early death.

Of course, I cannot deny that *some* nutrients are destroyed by cooking. This would include some of the B vitamins and vitamin C. Therefore it is best if your diet consists of a balanced combination of both raw and properly cooked foods in order to get the most nutrition all the way around. Just be sure than any raw fruits or vegetables you consume are washed first in order to prevent ingestion of any potential contaminants; this includes organically grown products.

SOY

Soy, a.k.a. soya products are made from soybeans, a popular Asian legume that is consumed as soy milk, tofu, toasted soy beans, edamame, natto, miso, tamari, tempeh, textured soy protein and textured vegetable protein. Soy is one of the few plant foods which contains sufficient amounts of all nine essential amino acids, meaning it is a complete protein food, making it a favorite among vegetarians and vegans.

Soy is well-known for containing substances called *isoflavones* – compounds known to have estrogenic effect, which means they behave like estrogen hormones in the body. Because isoflavones are plant based they are sometimes referred to as *phytoestrogens* (*phyto* = plant). Due to the isoflavones' estrogenic effect they readily attach to the estrogen receptors in breast tissue in direct competition to your own biological estrogen produced within your body. Because isoflavones have weaker estrogenic effect than your own biological estrogen, this is thought to be protective against breast cancer because the biological estrogen cannot attach to the receptors

123

which are already filled by the isoflavones. This is generally thought to be protective against estrogen-fueled breast cancers, yet there is still controversy as to whether this is really true.

Research has noted that Asian women, who tend to consume a much larger amount of dietary soy in their lifetimes, also have a much lower rate of breast cancers. Other research has noted that taking soy *supplements* (which are more concentrated than soy foods) tends to stimulate estrogen-responsive cancers. So, should soy products be avoided? One study published in 2001[421] stated in part of its conclusion:

> *"In regard to breast cancer, the isoflavones, specifically genistein, have paradoxical effects that can be resolved when you consider dosage and timing of administration. For example, prepubertal exposure to genistein appears to be protective against the development of breast cancer, but the consumption of the phytoestrogen in either pure form or in soy protein isolate, after development of an estrogen-dependent breast cancer may enhance the growth of that tumor as determined by this study."*

In short, it was noted that soy exposure *before* the onset of puberty appeared to protect against estrogen-dependent breast cancer, but soy exposure *after* having already *developed* such a cancer may fuel the existing cancer further. The study further noted that, even though soy may help protect against heart disease and lower cholesterol, post-menopausal women who are at risk of developing breast cancer should use caution when it comes to consuming soy products and supplements.

Other studies recorded similar findings,[422] [423]strongly suggesting that lifelong soy consumption before developing breast cancer is protective, while consumption *during* hormone-dependent breast cancer may be harmful. As for consumption of soy *after* the cancer has been beaten, a study involving 1,954 breast cancer patients showed that those who consumed soy at normal Asian dietary levels had fewer recurrences of breast cancer than those who consumed less soy. This was especially true of women who were taking the estrogen-blocking medication tamoxifen after treatment.[424] In a pooled analysis of 9,514 breast cancer patients it was found that patients who consumed approximately 10mg of soy isoflavones per day saw a significant reduction in breast cancer recurrence.[425]

So what does this mean? It means that, for patients who *do not* have an *active* estrogen-fueled cancer, normal dietary consumption of soy is likely safe, though each individual circumstance may vary. I strongly recommend eating no more than three servings of soy products per day and discontinue taking soy supplements (because

421 *Soy Diets Containing Varying Amounts of Genistein Stimulate Growth of Estrogen-Dependent (MCF-7) Tumors in a Dose Dependent Manner* (Clinton D. Allred, 2001)

422 *Is Soy Consumption Good or Bad for the Breast?* (Hilakivi-Clarke, 2010)

423 *Soy food Intake during Adolescence and Subsequent Risk of Breast Cancer among Chinese Women"* Xiao Ou Shu, 2001)

424*Soy Isoflavones and Risk of Cancer Recurrence in a Cohort of Breast Cancer Survivors: Life After Cancer Epidemiology (LACE) Study* (Guha, 2009)

425*Soy food intake after diagnosis of breast cancer and survival: an in-depth analysis of combined evidence from cohort studies of US and Chinese women* (Nechuta, 2012)

supplements contain much higher levels of isoflavones than that of a normal diet). Absolutely speak with your physicians and holistic health practitioners regarding your individual circumstance before continuing with any soy in your diet if you are at risk for estrogen-fueled cancers.

VEGAN DIET

Many people, including myself, advocate for vegan eating. A vegan diet consists solely of plant-based products, forgoing all animal and dairy foods.[426] Not only does a vegan diet offer plenty of fiber, nutrients, and heart-healthy fats but it also eliminates excess cholesterol from your diet.[427] Vegan diets also lower your risk of heart disease, and obesity, *and,* because animal proteins tend to elevate levels of IGF-1[428] – a growth hormone implicated in the growth of cancer – vegan diets are known to lower the risk of developing cancer.

A large study involving more than 69,000 participants reported that vegans have lower rates of cancer than both meat-eaters and vegetarians.[429] Vegan women, for example, had 34 percent lower rates of female-specific cancers such as breast, cervical, and ovarian cancer in comparison to those whose diets included animal proteins. Although vegetarians experienced a lower risk of gastrointestinal cancers than the meat eaters, the vegan subjects showed a significant decrease in female cancers overall.

Vegan diets are just as healthy for men when it comes to cancer risk. One study involving 696 male participants observed that IGF-1[430] was, on the average, 9% lower in vegan men than in meat-eating men and 8% lower than in vegetarian men.[431] Since earlier research has noted that men who had an 8% increase in IGF-1 tended to develop prostate cancer,[432] it is clear that the 9% decrease in vegan men is a significant factor in lowering the risk.

Another study, experimenting on prostate cancer cells, showed that the blood of men who consumed a vegan diet for a year has eight times more killing power against the cancer cells than men who ate a standard American diet.[433] Encouraged by this find, experiments were performed on ER+ and PR+ breast cancer cells. Researchers found that the blood of women who consumed a plant-based diet for only 14 days also showed a significant reduction in cancer cells growth.[434] Clearly, a plant based diet is a vital part of fighting your cancer.

Even if you've *already* developed cancer it is not too late to start eating a

---

426 This is in contrast to a vegetarian diet, which allows dairy, eggs, and honey.

427 A healthy body manufactures all the cholesterol you need for your system, you do not need to obtain more from your diet.

428 "IGF-1" is also known as Insulin-like Growth Factor.

429 *Vegetarian diets and the incidence of cancer in a low-risk population* (Tantamango-Bartley, 2013)

430 Insulin-like Growth Factor 1, implicated in the development of some cancers.

431 *Hormones and Diet: Low Insulin-like Growth Factor-1 but Normal Bioavailable Androgens in Vegan Men.* (Allen, 2000)

432 *Growth Hormone and Prostate Cancer: Guilty by Association?* (Grimberg, 1999)

433 *Intensive lifestyle changes may affect the progression of prostate cancer.* (Ornish, 2005)

434 *Effects of a low-fat, high-fiber diet and exercise program on breast cancer risk factors in vivo and tumor cell growth and apoptosis in vitro.* (Barnard, 2006)

vegan diet now. Switching to a vegan diet now will give you significant anti-cancer benefits such as:

- Immediate decrease in your IGF-1 levels, thus depriving tumors of the growth hormone.
- Reduced diet-based inflammation due to reduced intake in saturated fats.
- It is gentler on your digestive system, which may help reduce the nausea and vomiting associated with some chemotherapy agents.
- Reduced risk of developing other cancers later in life.

Chapter 9
HOLISTIC HORMONE THERAPY

Hormone therapy is not the same as hormone replacement therapy ("HRT"). Hormone replacement therapy is when a person is prescribed artificial hormones to replace the natural hormones that are not being manufactured in the body (such as during menopause). *Hormone therapy*, by contrast, is a system of treatment which *suppresses* the body's natural manufacture of hormones as a way of weakening hormone-fueled cancers (prostate, testicle, breast, endometrial a.k.a. uterine, ovarian, and some kidney cancers). Because hormone therapy merely weakens the cancerous cells it is usually paired with chemotherapy agents and/or radiation treatments which actively destroy the cells. The type of treatment that a patient will require depends upon the type of cancer, if it has spread and how far, and if the patient has other health problems. Hormone-fueled cancers are a little different from other cancers because these require the presence of certain hormones in order to grow. Because the hormones help feed the cancer's growth a patient needs to starve the cancer of the hormone in order gain control. Let me explain how this works:

In order to maintain a healthy system your body needs certain hormones to act on certain cells in order to maintain your gender-specific traits. These hormones are testosterone, progesterone, and estrogen. Although everyone has all of these hormones in their bodies gender differences dictate how high or low the levels of these hormones are that course through our veins. For example, men need higher levels of testosterone to deepen their voices, grow facial hair, and to make healthy sperm cells. In contrast, women need higher levels of estrogen in order to achieve their feminine curves and induce healthy egg production in their ovaries.

In order for these hormones to work in our bodies they need to be collected by certain body cells which are specially equipped to receive these hormones. This special "equipment" is known as hormone receptors, which are located on the outer membranes of these cells in order to more easily assimilate the hormones flowing past in the blood stream. Let me give you an example of how this works:

A healthy breast cell in a female needs estrogen in order to be stimulated to reproduce, thereby creating and maintaining the female breasts; therefore a breast cell has estrogen receptors on its surface. When estrogen molecules in the blood stream flow over the cell the molecules fit into the cell's receptors much like a key fits into a lock. When the cell receives enough estrogen in its receptors these "keys" activate the cell to begin reproduction. A healthy cell will reproduce a certain number of times before dying, after which it will be replaced with other "newborn" cells. This is normal and usual and the way it should be. *However*, if a breast cell begins mutating to the point of being cancerous, this becomes a serious problem because cancer cells have lost their ability to die. Therefore, a breast cancer cell will still receive the "grow signals" from estrogen molecules, yet it will not die no matter how many times it reproduces. And, since cells basically clone themselves during reproduction, this one cancer cell will be producing only more cancer cells, which also will not die. As the numbers of these cancer cells increase, the more they are fueled by "grow signals" from the body's natural cycle of estrogen release. Therefore, the best way to stop this particular group of cancer cells is to inhibit their growth by starving them of estrogenic hormones while you use chemotherapy and/or radiation treatments to actively kill them. Hormone therapy can accomplish this starvation in one of three ways : **(1)** The therapeutic agent can fill the receptors on the cancer cell surfaces, effectively blocking the hormone "keys" from fitting into the cell. **(2)** The therapeutic agent can decrease or eliminate the body's production of the hormone altogether, preventing the "keys" for the receptors from existing. **(3)** The therapeutic agent may be *another* hormone which slows or stops the growth of the cancer.

When a cancer is fueled by hormones it is known as a hormone positive cancer, which includes estrogen receptor positive (a.k.a. ER+) and progesterone receptor positive (a.k.a. PR+) cancers. If the cancer cells lack receptors for these hormones they are then regarded as negative (ER- and PR-). Some cancers may feature both kinds of receptors and some may feature only one. The oncologist will order tests to discover which, if any, receptors the cancer has in order to create the best treatment plan for you. If your cancer does not test positive for either receptor then it is considered a hormone-negative cancer, which means hormone-suppressing treatments will not be necessary.

Women are not the only ones who can develop hormone-fueled cancers – it can sometimes be a problem for men too. For example, prostate cancer tends to be associated with testosterone and other androgens, while testicular cancer can be associated with androgens *or* HCG[435] and estrogen. The oncologist will order tests to discover which receptors, if any, the cancer has in order to create the best treatment plan for you.

One thing to be aware of during hormone therapy is that the therapeutic agent does not know the difference between a healthy cell and a cancerous cell. Therefore, this hormonal treatment is universal throughout your body which means your healthy cells are also deprived of the hormone, and this may cause certain side effects. Depending upon the hormone therapy used, this may include side effects such as:
For men and women: Hot flashes, loss of libido, nausea, and fatigue.
For women: Changes in the menstrual cycle, vaginal dryness, and mood swings.
For men: Breast growth, weakened bones, weight gain, and diarrhea.

HOLISTIC INFORMATION
When a patient is facing a hormone-fueled cancer he or she needs to be aware that some foods, supplements, and herbs may encourage production of certain hormones and this may work against the physician-prescribed treatment plan. Knowing which foods and substances to avoid is an important factor in ensuring your treatment plan works better for you.

---

435 HCG = Human Chorionic Gonadotropin , a hormone usually associated with pregnant females.
    Men with this particular type of cancer will test positive for pregnancy if this hormone is present.

Androgen/Testosterone Fueled Cancers:

Treatment for these cancers involves suppressing the androgens[436] responsible for the cancer. Androgens are made primarily in the testicles, however the adrenal glands, which sit atop your kidneys, also produce small amounts of androgens in both men and women. If you are on a treatment plan to reduce your levels of androgens be aware that any herb or supplement used for increasing muscle mass or enhancing sexual performance will act like androgens in your body. Since these will work directly against your prescribed treatment plan you need to avoid these plants which are known to increase androgen levels. Examples of items to avoid include (but are not limited to): Epimedium spp.,[437] fenugreek (*Trigonella foenum-graecum*),[438] galangal (*Alpinia galangal*), rooiwortel (*Bulbine natalensis*), tongkat ali (*Eurycoma longifolia*)[439] and tackweed (*Tribulus terrestris*).[440]

Estrogen Fueled Cancers:

Estrogen is produced mainly in the female's ovaries however it is also produced in the brain, the adrenal glands, and in the male's testicles. Although estrogen is usually viewed as a "female" hormone, both men and women can develop estrogen-fueled cancers. If you are on a treatment plan to reduce your levels of estrogen be aware that some supplements, foods, and herbs contain plant-based estrogens (phytoestrogens) and mushroom-based estrogens (mycoestrogens).[441] Since these can work directly against your prescribed treatment plan you need to avoid them. Foods, herbs, and substances which are known to contain these estrogens include: alfalfa (*Medicago sativa*), American ginseng (*Panax quinquefolius*), animal milks, anise (*Pimpinella anisum*), Asian ginseng (*Panax ginseng*), black cohosh (*Actaea racemosa*), blessed thistle (*Cnicus benedictus*), blue cohosh (*Caulophyllum thalictroides*), chaste berry (*Vitex agnus-castus*), damiana (*Turnera diffusa*), dong quai (*Angelica sinensis*), evening primrose (*Oenothera spp.*), fennel (*Foeniculum vulgare*), flaxseed/linseed (*Linum usitatissimum*), ginkgo (*Ginkgo biloba*), kudzu (*Pueraria montana*), licorice (*Glycyrrhiza glabra*), red clover (*Trifolium pratense*), scaly wood mushroom (*Agaricus sylvaticus /Agaricus blazei*), sesame (*Sesamum indicum*), soy (*Glycine max*), sunflower seeds (*Helianthus spp*), wheat germ (*Triticum aestivum*), yams (*Dioscorea spp.*), and yarrow (*Achillea millefolium*). Also, avoid any commercial supplement designed for relieving menopause symptoms or enhancing sexual performance.

There is some controversy as to whether estrogen containing plants are actually strong enough to fuel one's cancer. In truth, phytoestrogens are much, *much* weaker than your own biological estrogens and therefore will not normally affect a

---

436 Androgen hormones include: Androstenedione (Andro), Dehydroepiandrosterone (DHEA), Dihydrotestosterone, and testosterone

437 Epimedium plants contain icariin, a substance which acts similar to testosterone. Common name for these plants are "horny goat weed." "bishop's hat," "fairy wings" and "yin yang huo."

438 Contains fenuside, a.k.a. testofen, substance which acts similar to testosterone.

439 Common name "Long Jack." Contains androgenic quassinoids.

440 A.k.a. puncture vine. Contains an androgenic substance known as protodioscin.

441 Isoflavones are among the most commonly found phytoestrogens.

healthy person so long as the plant is not concentrated into a supplement. Often times, in their non-concentrated levels, these weaker estrogens can fill in the estrogen receptors on cells thus blocking the stronger biological estrogens from taking hold; this is actually protective against developing future estrogen-fueled cancers. However, when consumers begin to buy *concentrated* products, such as commercial supplements and tinctures, this is when the problems may appear because these concentrated levels move closer to the strengths seen in your body's natural estrogens. Moderation is key, therefore I do not recommend over-processed, concentrated products for *anyone* without your physician's supervision.

As for patients who are *currently fighting* an estrogen-fueled cancer I advise that you avoid all substances containing phytoestrogens until you are cleared of your cancer. To lower the risk of your biological estrogens causing your cancer to recur (reappear) after your treatments have finished it is suggested that you consume up to three servings of non-concentrated phytoestrogen products daily to displace the biological estrogens in your cell receptors. Be sure to speak with your oncologist to discuss if this plan is right for you. One large study involving 5,042 female breast cancer survivors observed that women who consume soy-based foods in moderation after breast cancer have a significantly decreased risk of death and recurrence.[442]

If you are currently fighting an estrogen-fueled cancer is also important to know that vegetables in the brassica/ cabbage family contain substances which tend to lower estrogen levels, so I encourage you to consume these several times per week (see the subheading "Brassica/Cruciferous Vegetables" in chapter 6 of this book). If you are allergic to brassicas, or simply do not like them, you may opt to speak to your oncologist and an experienced herbalist regarding the use of Rooiwortel (*Bulbine natalensis*),[443] a folk herb from the southern regions of the African continent. Although rooiwortel is usually employed for improving testosterone levels studies have found that this herb also significantly lowers blood levels of estrogen in male lab rats (though there were not as significant a decrease of estrogen found in the female rats).[444] Caution must be considered though; studies have also shown that therapeutic levels of this herb risks damage to the liver and kidneys[445] and may also increase white blood cell counts.[446]

Progesterone Fueled Cancers:

Progesterone is a steroid hormone that is produced in the uterine lining, adrenal glands, ovaries, and the placenta. This hormone is the starting point for the manufacture of estrogens in the body. Although progesterone is not found in the plant

---

442 *Soy Food Intake and Breast Cancer Survival"* (Xiao Ou Shu, 2009)

443 Also known by the names "Ibhucu: and "Ingcelwane."

444 *Reproductive toxicologic evaluations of Bulbine natalensis Baker stem extract in albino rats.* (Yakubu, 2009)

445 *Effect of Bulbine natalensis Baker stem extract on the functional indices and histology of the liver and kidney of male Wistar rats.* (Afolayan, 2009)

446 *Effect of aqueous extract of Bulbine natalensis Baker stem on haematological and serum lipid profile of male Wistar rats.* (Yakubu, 2009)

kingdom there are several plants which contain certain sterols (a.k.a. phytosterols)[447] and these sterols are chemically similar to progesterone. As a result, when you consume these sterols your body uses them for the synthesis of progesterone thus these can act similar to progesterone when consumed. If you are on a treatment plan to reduce your levels of progesterone be aware that the following plants sources are high in sterols which may increase your progesterone levels: alfalfa (*Medicago sativa*), American ginseng (*Panax quinquefolius*), ashwagandha (*Withania somnifera*), Asian ginseng (*Panax ginseng*), asparagus (*Asparagus officinalis*), beta carotene[448], borage (*Borago officinalis*), chaste berry (*Vitex agnus-castus*), chocolate, crêpe ginger (*Cheilocostus speciosus*), damiana (*Turnera diffusa*), dragon's beard[449] (*Ophiopogon japonicus*), evening primrose (*Oenothera spp.*), fenugreek (*Trigonella foenum-graecum*), horse chestnut (*Aesculus hippocastanum*), Kenya Oak (*Vitex keniensis*), licorice (*Glycyrrhiza glabra*), oregano (*Origanum vulgare*), rapeseed/rapaseed (*Brassica napus*), red clover (*Trifolium pratense*), sarsaparilla (*Smilax ornata*), schisandra (*Schisandra chinensis*), sesame seeds (*Sesamum indicum*), soapwort (*Saponaria officinalis*), soybeans (*Glycine max*), sunflower seeds (*Helianthus spp.*), thyme (*Thymus vulgaris*), turmeric (*Curcuma longa*), unpasteurized milks, vegetable oils (including margarine), and verbena (*Verbena officinalis*).

Tandem Estrogen and Progesterone Fueled Cancers:

Some patients develop a cancer that tests positive for both estrogen and progesterone receptors. In these cases speak to your oncologist and holistic practitioners about the guidelines in this chapter for both types of hormones so he or she can create a treatment plan that works all the way around.

HORMONE-BASED PRESCRIPTIONS

Many people are prescribed hormone-based medications for a number of reasons such as birth control, excessive acne, endocrine disorders, erectile dysfunction, fertility treatments, hormone replacement therapy, regulation of the menstrual cycle, vaginal lubrication, transgender maintenance, and other reasons. If you are dealing with a hormone-fueled cancer you absolutely must tell your oncologist if you are currently prescribed any kind of hormone-based medications from other doctors as these may interfere with your cancer treatment. Hormone based medications come in several forms:

- *Creams*: Estrogen creams, progesterone creams, and testosterone creams. This includes both topical formulas and formulas for internal use.
- *Gels*: These may contain estrogens, progesterones, or testosterones and includes both topical formulas and formulas for internal use.
- *Implants*: These can be pellets (available in Europe and Australia) or matchstick-sized rods inserted under the skin.

---

447 These sterols include diosgenin, saponins, and stigmasterol,
448 Natural sources of beta carotene include sweet potatoes, carrots, orange winter squashes, spinach, kale, cantaloupe, apricots, red sweet peppers, yams and peas.
449 Also known as: Mondograss, monkeygrass, snake's beard, and mai men dong

- *Injections*: These include injections of testosterone, estrogen, or progesterone.
- *Inserts*: Vaginal rings, vaginal tablets, IUD's.
- *Patches*: Testosterone patches, birth control patches, and hormone replacement therapy patches.
- *Pills*: Hormone-containing tablets, usually used for HRT, regulation of the menstrual cycle, or birth control.
- *Suppositories*: Creams, foams, or gels designed to be inserted into the vagina

If you are unsure whether your medications are hormone-based do not hesitate to ask your prescribing physician or your oncologist.

Chapter 10
HEAT THERAPY

Heat therapy (also known as thermal therapy, hyperthermia, or thermotherapy) is a treatment which uses heat to promote health and healing. Although this type of therapy has many applications this chapter will focus on its applications in cancer treatment.

Research shows that cancer cells are much more susceptible to destruction from heat than healthy cells are, [450] [451] and some studies have found that heat therapy significantly increases the effectiveness of alkylating agents, platinums, taxanes, vinca alkaloids, and other chemotherapy agents.[452] In 2006 a German study was published which showed heat therapy helped reduce metastatic tumors in breast cancer patients, even to the point of actual remission in some cases.[453] An Italian study published in 2010 stated that heat therapy should be viewed as the fourth pillar in the treatment of cancer alongside surgery, chemotherapy, and radiotherapy.[454]

Heat therapy can be performed using controlled microwaves, radio waves, infrared light, magnetic waves, heated water, or sound waves depending upon the location(s) of the tumor(s). According to the Italian study mentioned above, heat treatment boosts the effectiveness of chemotherapy medications because it increases the absorption of the medications directly into the cancer cells themselves; this is good information for a patient whose cancer is becoming resistant to chemotherapy medications. Another study supports this, showing that breast cancer patients who were treated with heat therapy along with chemotherapy had significantly better responses to the chemotherapy agents used.[455]

Heat therapy is best given either immediately before or immediately after radiation therapy and chemotherapy in order to amplify sensitization of the tumor(s). Since heat therapy has been shown to be a very effective weapon against cancer, let's take a closer look at the different ways this treatment is administered:

LOCAL HYPERTHERMIA, a.k.a. *"thermal ablation,"*[456] uses very high temperatures (up to 212°F or 100°C) directly aimed at the tumor itself and is usually intended for tumors that are no larger than 2 inches across (5cm).

---

450 *Physical principles of local heat therapy for cancer.* (Babbs, 1981)

451 Book: **Cancer Treatment – Conventional and Innovative Approaches** "Chapter 12: Hyperthermia – Cancer Treatment and Beyond" pp.257-283 Ahmed Bettaieb, et al [Book edited by Leticia Rangel] This is an "open access" book available online.

452 *Hyperthermia in Combined Treatment of Cancer.* (Wust, 2002)

453 **23ʳᵈ Annual Meeting of the European Society for Hyperthermic Oncology**, May 27, 2006 "*Whole Body Hyperthermia in Patients With Breast Cancer and Painful Metastasis*" A Herzog et al

454 *he Role of Hyperthermia in the Battle Against Cancer* (Palazzi, 2010)

455 **Clinical Cancer Research**, Feb.2002, Vol.8, pp.374-382 "*Liposomal Doxorubicin in Conjunction with Re-irradiation and Local Hyperthermia Treatment in Recurrent Breast Cancer, A Phase I/II Trial*" Vassilios E. Kouloulias, et al

456 Ablation: Surgical destruction of diseased tissue usually through heating, abrading, evaporating, or freezing.

Local hyperthermia works by heating the tumor cells to death while also destroying the tumor's associated blood vessels. If the targeted tumor is near the surface of the skin the oncologist may use a specialized heat machine aimed at the location. If the tumor is deeper in the tissues he or she will likely opt for using a specialized probe, called a thermocouple, which features a tip that can be inserted directly into the tumor and heated – you will be given a local anesthetic before the thermocouple is inserted. During treatment the technologist will continually monitor the temperatures in and around the tumor to ensure safe, effective treatment. Because it can take as long as one hour to complete treatment from set-up to finish you should be sure to use the restroom before starting. Heating methods usually use radio-frequency, ultrasound, or microwaves as the source. Some patients may feel mildly uncomfortable heat sensations during treatment; do not be shy about telling the technologist if this happens to you as he or she can adjust the treatment if necessary. There is a likelihood that some scarring may result after treatment dependent upon the size of the tumor, but this is a small price to pay. Remember, few warriors win a battle without sustaining a few battle scars.

REGIONAL HYPERTHERMIA uses lower heat temperatures (up to 113°F or 45°C) aimed at a region of the body instead of narrowing down to just the tumor itself. This may involve an entire organ, limb, or body cavity. This is usually applied toward cancers which have produced a large tumor. Because of the broad area it covers it is not feasible to use the higher temperatures that are employed in local hyperthermia. Due to the temperatures being lower the cancer cells are not directly destroyed, however they are weakened enough to become significantly vulnerable to chemotherapy and radiation treatments. Because there are many variables regarding location and size of tumors there are several ways in which to perform this treatment which runs the gamut from specialized heat treating machines to surgery under general anesthesia. Because each patient's situation is unique I strongly advise you to speak with your oncologist regarding the method of treatment that will work best for *you*.

WHOLE BODY HYPERTHERMIA also uses low heat similar to regional hyperthermia, only in this kind of treatment your *entire body* is being treated, not just parts of it. This type of treatment is commonly used when metastasis has occurred and many different body parts need to be treated simultaneously. Patients undergoing this type of hyperthermia will often be treated through the use of warming blankets, warm water immersion, or a thermal chamber. The general effect is to give the body an artificial fever in order to weaken the cancerous cells to increase their vulnerability.

Although heat therapy is a proven, effective treatment, patients need to receive this treatment only under the care of a licensed physician or a properly trained holistic practitioner in order to reduce the risk of patient injury. Although heat is a natural form of energy this treatment is not without risks. Before starting heat therapy you must be sure your oncologist or practitioner is aware of any of the following:

- If you have a pacemaker, vagal stimulator, pins, plates, or other implanted device as some heating methods may affect these items.
- If you are on any medications which reduce pain or may induce drowsiness or dizziness.
- If you have any blood clotting or bleeding issues
- If you have a history of stroke or heart attack
- If you have had surgery in the past 72 hours
- If you have compromised pain response
- If you have circulations problems
- If you are pregnant

Aside from the above-mentioned contraindications, you should also be aware of the possible side effects you may experience during your course of heat treatments. Let your oncologist know if you experience any of the following:

- *Localized Heat Therapy:* Pain, infection, bleeding, blood clots, open sores, swelling, blistering, burns, nerve or tissue damage.
- *Regional or Whole Body Heat Therapy*: Nausea or vomiting, diarrhea, redness, blistering, swelling, heart arrhythmia, circulation issues.

You should also know that, on occasion, you may have an underlying health condition that you weren't already aware of; in such cases heat therapy may intensify those conditions. These conditions may include emphysema, COPD, asthma, circulatory issues, and more. Please be sure to discuss these risks with your doctor before making any decisions for heat treatment.

One more thing that should be mentioned is the fact that heat-treated cancer cells can become heat resistant in some cases if the heat treatment sessions are scheduled too close together. This means that if you want hyperthermia to work for you, then you will need to go according to the schedule of the person(s) responsible for your treatment. Demanding extra sessions of treatments through either your cancer center or your holistic practitioner may actually hurt you instead of help you. This risk of heat resistance is also another reason why your oncologist *and* holistic practitioners need to know all of your treatments: If one does not know that the other is performing heat therapy treatments on you he or she may unknowingly recommend further heat treatments which could lead to your cancer's resistance.

Chapter 11
HYDRAZINE SULFATE

Hydrazine sulfate (a.k.a. Sehydrin) is a low-cost nutritional supplement found in locations which sell vitamins, herbs, and supplements. It is a monoamine oxidase inhibitor (MAOI), which means it must not be taken concurrently with other MAOI's, tranquilizers, benzodiazepines, barbituates, alcohol, or other central nervous system depressant medications as these will block its effectiveness. Check with your prescribing physicians if you are unsure whether any of your medications fall into those categories. Individuals using hydrazine sulfate must also avoid foods which contain tyramine, a natural substance in some foods[457] which can interact with MAOI's, resulting in dangerously increased blood pressure.

Many holistic practitioners regard hydrazine sulfate as a powerful agent to reverse cachexia and reduce the size of cancerous tumors. It is thought that hydrazine sulfate works by blocking the liver enzymes needed for synthesizing glucose, a form of sugar preferred by cancer cells to create energy. Blocking this production of glucose essentially starves the tumor and decreases its size as well as reducing the tumor-induced cachexia. The problem is that, due to conflicts in clinical trial results there seems to be a lot of confusion as to whether hydrazine sulfate actually works. Therefore, in the interest of putting the confusion to rest this chapter will discuss the clinical trials and what it means to cancer patients.

Hydrazine sulfate as a cancer treatment came to light in the 1960's when Dr. Joseph Gold, director of the Syracuse Cancer Research Center in Syracuse, NY, pioneered its use for cancer treatment. His ideas came from the work of Nobel prize winner Dr. Otto Warburg who posited that cancer cells obtained their energy through the metabolism of glucose; subsequent research supported Warburg's ideas.[458] [459] According to Dr. Gold, hydrazine sulfate treatment works best when patients avoid the use of alcohol (including alcohol in cooking, over-the-counter medications, home remedies, etc.), barbituates, benzodiazepines, and antidepressants during treatment due to the fact that those medications interfere with its efficacy. He also noted that dosage is also important, as too high a dose of hydrazine sulfate can create a toxicity that shortens patients' life spans. Dr. Gold performed in vivo testing with laboratory rats which seemed to indicate that treatment with the substance inhibited tumor

---

457 Foods which contain tyramine include aged meats, almonds, Asian sauces, avocados, bananas, beef or chicken liver, beer, broad beans, cheese (including cottage cheese), chocolate, coffee, cured meats, dried fruits, fermented or pickled foods, herring, meat tenderizers, monosodium glutamate (MSG), peanuts, pineapple, pumpkin seeds, raisins, sesame seeds, smoked foods, snow peas, sour cream, soy products, wine, yeast extracts (including brewer's yeast), yogurt, and other foods. Consult with your physician or a registered dietitian for a complete list.

458 *Oxygen Consumption and Glycolysis of Human Malignant and Normal Tissue (* MacBeth, 1962)

459 *Metabolic Profiles in Human Solid Tumors. 1. A New Technic for the Utilization of Human Solid Tumors in Cancer Research and Its Application to the Anaerobic Glycolysis of Isologous Benign and Malignant Colon Tissues (Gold, 1966)*

growth.[460] This encouraged him to move on to human clinical trials, in which he found that 70% of the test subjects in one trial experienced increased appetite, weight gain, and strength with a decrease in pain, while 17% of the test subjects in the trial also experienced tumor regression.[461] Due to these results Dr. Gold recommended that hydrazine sulfate be used as a concurrent treatment with conventional cancer therapies. This idea is supported by the following clinical trial published by a different team of researchers:

This clinical trial involved 65 non-small-cell lung cancer patients in advanced stages of the disease. The purpose was to evaluate the effects of hydrazine sulfate on the progression of the disease. This trial was performed as a randomized, prospective, double-blind, placebo-controlled study. Both the control group and the experimental group received six cycles of chemotherapy – radiotherapy was not permitted. Patients were evaluated at the start of each chemotherapy cycle by clinical examination and chest x-ray imaging. Monthly dietary counseling was also incorporated in order to promote weight maintenance – all dietary intake was oral (i.e. no tube feedings or parenteral feedings). This study found that patients who received the hydrazine sulfate treatments had a higher survival rate and increase in weight gain than those who received the placebo. However, the study also found that, although tumor size did decrease somewhat during treatment, the decrease in the hydrazine sulfate treated patients was not significantly different from the placebo treated patients.[462]

In a different clinical trial, performed by the Harbor-UCLA Medical Center, 38 advanced-stage cancer patients with cachexia symptoms were studied. Types of cancer in this study included non-small-cell lung cancers, gastric cancers, and breast cancers, among others. This was a randomized, placebo-controlled, double-blind study to evaluate hydrazine sulfate's effect on cachexia. Patients were given metabolic evaluations before commencing the study; chemotherapy patients had been at least four weeks since their last chemotherapy treatments (though 25 of the participants began chemotherapy treatments once the study was started). Evaluations were repeated 30 days after the start of hydrazine sulfate treatment and assessed. Participants who were using the hydrazine sulfate were gradually increased in dosage until reaching 60mg three times daily before meals. Compared to the placebo group, those using the test drug were shown to experience significant improvement in glucose tolerance and a significant decrease in total glucose production.[463]

Later, a Russian review regarding the efficacy of hydrazine sulfate in clinical trials looked at a total of 740 patients gleaned from research studies involving many different kinds of cancers. This pool of patients included those who had a history of chemotherapy, radiation therapy, surgery, and/or hormone therapy. Treatment

460 *inhibition of Walker 256 Intramuscular Carcinoma in Rats by Administration of Hydrazine Sulfate* (Gold, 1971)

461 *Use of hydrazine sulfate in terminal and preterminal cancer patients: results of investigational new drug (IND) study in 84 evaluable patients* (Gold, 1975)

462 *Hydrazine Sulfate Influence on Nutritional Status and Survival in Non-small-cell Lung Cancer* (Chlebowski, 1990)

463 *Influence of Hydrazine Sulfate on Abnormal Carbohydrate Metabolism In Cancer Patients With Weight Loss* (Chlebowski, 1984)

regimens in these studies were performed from 30-45 days per cycle with 2-6 weeks break in between cycles, depending upon the individual studies. Patients' use of alcohol and barbituates was prohibited during the cycles of hydrazine sulfate treatment during these studies. Out of the 740 patients involved, 374 of them (50%) achieved moderate to significant reduction in cachexia, with the best results showing in patients with recurrent desmosarcoma, fibrosarcoma, neuroblastoma, endometrial cancer, breast cancer, and Hodgkin's disease. [464]

A single case study[465] published by the Syracuse Cancer Research Center in 1999 also showed positive results: A 65 year old male diagnosed with large cell cancer of the lung was found to have residual cancer one month after a prior round of chemotherapy treatment. He began treatment with radiation, carboplatin, and hydrazine sulfate at 60mg three times daily. Within three months the patient gained 40 lbs (18kg) and was able to return to his place of employment. Although no sign of disease was found in his lung at the three month mark tests revealed metastasis in on of his adrenal glands, which was removed. At the time the case study was published the patient was still alive more than 8 years after removing the metastasis, meaning he achieved complete response ("CR" in cancer language).

These are not the only clinical trials and case studies showing positive results; there are plenty more, but I think the point is clear: Hydrazine sulfate has shown very encouraging results over the past few decades. In spite of this, however, there are many who believe that hydrazine sulfate doesn't really work at all. This is primarily due to a trio of clinical trials sponsored by the National Cancer Institute (NCI), the largest organization in the world funding cancer research with a budget set by the United States Congress.

The NCI sponsored three clinical trials which studied the effects of hydrazine sulfate on cancer patients. Each of these trials were randomized, placebo-controlled, double-blind studies, and the results were published in the *Journal of Clinical Oncology* in June, 1994. One of these studies, involving 127 advanced-stage colorectal cancer patients, showed a lower survival rate, lower quality of life, and no difference in appetite or weight gain among the hydrazine sulfate users.[466] The second study, involving 266 patients with non-small-cell lung cancer, showed a negligible difference in survival rates, and no differences in appetite or weight changes. It also noted an increase in sensory and motor neuropathy in the hydrazine sulfate users.[467] In the third study, involving 243 non-small-cell lung cancer patients, results showed the hydrazine sulfate users experiencing worsening disease progression and decreased survival times compared to the placebo users.[468] These three studies are in complete

---

464 *Results of Clinical Evaluation of Hydrazine Sulfate* (Filov, 1990) (Using the English translation; original article written in Russian)

465 *Long Term Complete Response in Patient with Advanced Localized NSCLC with Hydrazine Sulfate, Radiation and Carboplatin, Refractory to Combination Chemotherapy* (Gold, 1999)

466 *"Randomized Placebo-controlled Evaluation of Hydrazine Sulfate in Patients With Advanced Colorectal Cancer* (Loprinzi, 1994)

467 *Cisplatin, Vinblastine, and Hydrazine Sulfate in Advanced Non-small-cell Lung Cancer: A Randomized Placebo-controlled, Double-bling Phase III Study of the Cancer and Leukemia Group B* (Kosty, 1994)

468 *Placebo-controlled Trial of Hydrazine Sulfate in Patients With Newly Diagnosed Non-small-cell*

contrast to the aforementioned studies – what happened?

When these NCI-sponsored studies became public proponents in favor of hydrazine sulfate heavily objected, resulting in a government investigation into the matter. Although the final report decided the NCI-sponsored studies *"were not flawed"*, the actual contents of the report confirm the truth of the matter. Part of the report states *"In testing hydrazine sulfate, NCI permitted study patients to use tranquilizing agents, barbituates, and alcohol in one NCI-sponsored clinical trial. In the other two trials, NCI prohibited the use of barbituates and alcohol, but patients were permitted to use tranquilizing agents as antiemetics to control nausea and vomiting."* This is important because, as mentioned earlier, patients using hydrazine sulfate should *not* be using tranquilizers, barbituates, or alcohol. The report also goes on to state that there were lapses in record-keeping and that the NCI did not require the completion of accurate records in at least one of the trials. The report also reveals that the NCI ignored cautions from the FDA regarding recommendations to avoid the use of tranquilizers and other contraindicated substances. How extensive was patient use of these contraindicated substances during these trials? According to the report, one of the studies allowed 88% of the test subjects to use benzodiazepine while 71% were allowed to use other tranquilizing agents, and another one of the studies showed that 78% of the test subjects used serotonin antagonist medications.[469] Although the report stopped short of defining the NCI-sponsored studies as "flawed", it is clear the studies were compromised by the inclusion of substances that are contraindicated.

As you can see, the perceived contradiction in studies is really a matter of which studies adhered to the proper recommendations. However, this does not mean you should go out and buy yourself some hydrazine sulfate and start consuming it. As with all other medications, there are some serious considerations to discuss with your health care team before using this treatment:

1. Although hydrazine sulfate is an over-the-counter substance, do not take it without the supervision of your oncologist due to several possible contraindications and risk of side effects. You need to keep in mind that just because it works for many doesn't mean it works for *all*. Not only are certain medications incompatible with the substance, but certain health conditions are also contraindicated. The following health issues must be considered if you are deciding whether to take hydrazine sulfate: Pregnancy, breastfeeding, liver disease, diabetes, impending surgery, and use of certain other medications. Side effects can include nausea and vomiting, dizziness, drowsiness, nerve damage, behavioral changes, restlessness, seizures, confusion, breathing irregularities, blood sugar changes, rash, kidney damage, and coma.

Lung Cancer (Loprinzi, 1994)

469 **United States General Accounting Office**, September 1995, GAO/HEHS-95-141 Hydrazine Sulfate *"Cancer Drug Research: Contrary to Allegation NIH Hydrazine Sulfate Studies Were Not Flawed"*

2. If your oncologist agrees that this may be a good treatment for you, do not take more than the amount he or she recommends as it can be toxic in too-large doses. Be sure to inform your oncologist of any side effects that may develop. Be sure your oncologist is also aware of any alternative treatments you are currently using.

3. Do not be discouraged if your results do not match someone else's; there are plenty of other therapies to help you get through your fight against cancer – many patients have done it, and so can you.

4. Be sure that your doctors and your practitioners are all aware that you are using this treatment.. They need to be informed so they can adjust your therapies, note any changes in your health, and keep in proper communication.

5. If, after careful consideration you choose to start using hydrazine sulfate, do not suddenly stop any medications or supplements you are already taking. Always seek the advice of your prescribing physicians and practitioners before starting treatment and before discontinuing use.

Chapter 12
MEDICINAL MUSHROOMS
Do not use medicinal mushrooms if you have any kind of mushroom allergy!

Medicinal mushrooms are known to be effective against cancer, however most of these tend to have antioxidants and immune-boosting properties which are contraindicated in certain cancer treatments. If your oncologist gives you the okay to use medicinal mushrooms you must also be aware that eating raw, whole mushrooms is not an effective method of administration. This is because the cell walls of mushrooms are very tough and simple chewing and digestion does not extract enough of the therapeutic agents to be absorbed into your system. Mushrooms need to be processed in such a way that the agents are preserved and yet able to be readily absorbed.[470] The following methods are preferable:

- *POWDERED*: Powdered mushroom preparations may come in capsule form or as a loose powder that can be added to foods and beverages. Do not add loose powder products to your foods until *after* your food has been already cooked, unless the instructions say otherwise.

- *FLUID*: Cold water extraction methods preserve metabolites, hot water extractions preserves the immune modulating properties, and alcohol (ethanol) extraction preserves antioxidants. Speak to your oncologist or a competent holistic practitioner regarding which extraction method is best for your treatment plan.

- *WHOLE, COOKED*: The only way to extract enough of the beneficial agents from the mushrooms is to either cook them or steep them in boiling water. They should be finely chopped and cooked only enough to soften them. Drink any broth that comes out from your cooked mushrooms. The fresher your mushrooms are the higher the level of therapeutic agents they contain.

ACTIVE HEXOSE CORRELATED COMPOUND

Also known as AHCC, this commercial formula produced in Japan is made from the extracts of medicinal mushrooms. It is marketed to be used concurrently with chemotherapy treatments as researchers believe it increases the activity of natural killer cells (a.k.a. "N.K."cells) in cancer patients. One study showed that AHCC helped reduce the risk of developing resistance to the chemotherapy agent gemcitabine in pancreatic cancer cells.[471] One in vivo study observed that AHCC boosted the efficacy of the chemotherapy agent 5-FU.[472] Another study showed that

---

470 Be aware that many medicinal mushroom extracts contain substances which are known to be toxic to your heart and blood cells when injected directly into the body. Therefore, do not receive mushroom products by injection if they were not originally intended or specially processed for that method of administration.

471 *Active Hexose-correlated Compound Down-regulates Heat Shock Factor 1, a Transcription Factor for HSP27, in Gemcitabine-resistant Human Pancreatic Cancer Cells.* (Tokunaga, 2015)

472*Active Hexose Correlated Compound Potentiates the Anti-tumor Effects of Low-dose 5-fluorouracil Through Modulation of Immune Function in Hepatoma 22 Bearing Mice.* (Z. Cao, 2015)

the use of AHCC can reduce changes in the sense of taste brought on by gemcitabine treatments.[473] One other study, using rats, found that using AHCC with the chemotherapy agents 6-mercaptopurine and methotrexate reduced hair loss and liver damage, and that using it with the agent cytosine arabinoside reduced hair loss.[474] One other study observed that AHCC can enhance the effects of cisplatin treatment while also reducing side effects such as kidney damage, bone marrow damage, and loss of appetite.[475] Doses as high as 6 grams daily have been established as safe for up to six months. Lower doses of 3 grams daily have been established as safe for up to nine years. *Precautions: Some patients have experienced side effects such as diarrhea and itching when taking this formula. This formula may decrease the effectiveness of the chemotherapy agent tamoxifen and others metabolized by the CYP2D6 enzyme, so be sure to check with your doctor before use.*

CHAGA MUSHROOM
Inonotus obliquus

This variety of this fungus grows primarily on birch trees. Birch trees produce a powerful anti-cancer substance known as betulinic acid in their bark; chaga mushrooms absorb this acid from the bark thus giving us easy access to the substance. Betulinic acid is an attractive agent because it is highly toxic to cancer cells without harming surrounding healthy cells. In vitro studies have shown that both water and ethanol extracts of chaga mushroom inhibit the growth of human colon cancer cells[476] [477] induces cell death in hepatoma cells,[478] and inhibits the growth of melanoma cells in mice.[479] Other mouse models showed that three weeks of oral dosing with chaga extract resulted in 60% tumor reduction and 25% reduction in metastatic nodules.[480] Chaga mushroom can be bought whole, as a powder, or as a tincture. When buying whole be sure to break it up into smaller chunks, dehydrate it for a few days, and then grind it into a powder. Allow the powder to dry for a few more days before sealing it for storage. Do not use temperatures above 125°F (51°C) while processing or storing this mushroom in order to preserve the betulinic acid. Mix 2 teaspoons (10ml) powder in one cup of very warm water, steep for 15 minutes, strain and drink. Use up to three

---

473 *Alleviating Effect of Active Hexose Correlated Compound (AHCC) on Chemotherapy-related Adverse Events in Patients with Unresectable Pancreatic Ductal Adenocarcinoma.* (Yanagimoto 2016)

474 *The Effect of Active Hexose Correlated Compound in Modulating Cytosine Arabinoside-induced Hair Loss, and 6-Mercaptopurine -and Methotrexate-induced Liver Injury in Rodents.* (Sun, 2009)

475 *The Influence of Active Hexose Correlated Compound (AHCC) on Cisplatin-evoked Chemotherapeutic and Side Effects in Tumor-bearing Mice.* (Hirose, 2007)

476 *Ethanol extract of Innotus obliquus (Chaga mushroom) induces G1 cell cycle arrest in HT-29 human colon cancer cells.* (H. S. Lee, 2015)

477 *Antitumor activity of water extract of a mushroom, Inonotus obliquus, against HT-29 human colon cancer cells.* (Sung Hak Lee, 2009)

478 *Chaga mushroom (Inonotus obliquus) Induces G0/G1 Arrest and Apoptosis in Human Hepatoma HepG2 Cells."* (Youn, 2008)

479 *Potential anticancer properties of the water extract of Inonotus [corrected] obliquus by induction of apoptosis in melanoma B16-F10 cells.* (Myung Ja Youn, 2009)

480 *Continuous intake of the Chaga mushroom (Inonotus obliquus) aqueous extract suppresses cancer progression and maintains body temperature in mice.* (Arata, 2016)

times daily. If using a commercial powder, extract, or tincture use according to package instructions. *Precautions: May contain oxalic acid do not take more than recommended amounts in order to reduce your risk of developing kidney stones. This product may thin your blood and may lower blood sugar. Do not harvest this mushroom without an expert mycologist (mushroom expert) to guide you as some similar looking mushrooms are very poisonous.*

CLOUD EAR FUNGUS
Auricularia Polytricha/ Auricularia auricula

This mushroom also goes by other names such as Jew's ear and Judas ear. It is commonly used as a culinary ingredient in Asian dishes, however in vitro studies have shown that substances in this mushroom are effective against certain types of human lung cancer by causing cell death.[481] To use, simply cook this mushroom in with your favorite cuisine. *Precautions: Thins the blood. May lower blood sugar levels.*

CORDYCEPS
Ophiocordyceps sinensis

A.k.a. Chinese caterpillar fungus, this fungus grows in ghost moth caterpillars and is found only in areas of Nepal and Tibet. Because of the scarcity of this fungus it is not commercially available and can be a costly treatment (though fees for treatment should not be exorbitant). Fortunately, a 2016 press release reported that Chinese researchers have developed a synthetic version of this fungus with a 97% DNA match to the natural product.[482] Studies have shown cordyceps to enhance the ability of cisplatin to inhibit the growth of non-small-cell lung cancer cells in vitro;[483] helps reverse low blood counts caused by the chemotherapy agent Taxol;[484] and has significant anti-cancer activity against oral cancers, liver cancer metastasis, and certain lung cancers. A substance in this fungus known as cordyceptin is also a powerful anti-inflammatory agent. However, a patient must not use this in concentrated form without trained guidance because this substance can also weaken the immune system and delay the healing of cuts and wounds. *Precautions: May lower blood sugar. May thin the blood.*

CRIMINI MUSHROOMS
Agaricus bisporus

Crimini mushrooms, a.k.a. baby bella mushrooms, are a common culinary ingredient. These mushrooms contain conjugated linoleic acid (CLA), a substance useful against ER+ breast cancers and colon cancer (see subheading "Conjugated

---

481 *Auricularia polytricha Polysaccharides Induce Cell Cycle Arrest and Apoptosis in Human Lung Cancer A549 Cells. (*JYu, 2014)

482 **Xinhua**, Editor: Xiang Bo, Sept. 10, 2016

483 *Polysaccharide of Cordyceps sinensis enhances cisplatin cytotoxicity in non-small cell lung cancer H157 cell line* (N. F. Ji, 2011)

484 *Cordyceps sinensis health supplement enhances recovery from taxol-induced leukopenia.* (Liu, 2008)

Linoleic Acid" in chapter 6 of this book for details). These mushrooms also have powerful anti-inflammatory properties. Simply cook these mushrooms in with your favorite cuisine. *Precautions: Patients with cardiovascular issues or diabetes should use caution when using products containing CLA. Side effects from CLA use include fatigue and digestive issues and may thin the blood.*

ENOKI
Flammulina velutipes
This mushroom, also known as enokitake, is a popular culinary ingredient. Japanese research noted that populations who consumed higher intakes of enoki mushrooms tended to have much lower rates of cancer than other populations. Specifically, in his studies he found that Japanese enoki farmers (who had the higher intakes) experienced 36% less cancers in men and 42% less cancer in the women. Further study led to the discovery that enoki mushrooms contain the proteins flammulin and proflamin, which have been shown to be effective against various types of cancers. More specific studies have shown enoki to be effective against certain liver cancer cells,[485] and ER+ and ER- breast cancer cells.[486] Simply cook the mushrooms in with your favorite cuisine. *Precautions: The raw form of this mushroom contains flammutoxin, a protein which is toxic to the heart, can stimulate an allergic response, and has strong action against blood cells, especially type O blood, when used as an injection. Flammutoxin is destroyed by heat (100 °F, or 37.7°C for 20 full minutes).*

MAITAKE
Grifola frondosa
A.k.a. Hen of the woods. This popular Japanese mushroom has been shown to have strong action against the metastasis of cancer through the body. Maitake D fraction, an extract from the maitake mushroom, is known to destroy cancer cells by causing cancer cell death and inhibits tumor blood vessel formation by reducing VEGF. In vitro studies have shown maitake to be effective against ER+ breast cancer cells,[487] enhances the effectiveness of dendritic cell therapy,[488] enhances interferon activity against bladder cells,[489] and inhibits the growth of four different lines of gastric cancer cells.[490] One other other study showed maitake to enhance the action of the chemotherapy agent cisplatin while reducing the risk of cisplatin-caused kidney

---

485 *Oral administration of an Enoki mushroom protein FVE activates innate and adaptive immunity and induces anti-tumor activity against murine hepatocellular carcinoma* (Chang, 2010)

486 *In vitro effects on proliferation, apoptosis and colony inhibition in ER-dependent and ER-independent human breast cancer cells by selected mushroom species."* (Y. H. Gu, 2006)

487 *Maitake (D fraction) mushroom extract induces apoptosis in breast cancer cells by BAK-1 gene activation.* (Soares, 2011)

488 *A polysaccharide extracted from Grifola frondosa enhances the anti-tumor activity of bone marrow-derived dendritic cell-based immunotherapy against murine colon cancer.* (Masuda, 2010)

489 *Synergistic potentiation of interferon activity with maitake mushroom d-fraction on bladder cancer cells* (Louie, 2010)

490 *Antitumor Effects of a Water-soluble Extract from Maitake (Grifola frondosa) on Human Gastric Cancer Cell Lines* (Shomori, 2009)

damage and bone marrow suppression.[491] Another study observed that the constituents in maitake promotes bone marrow repair after damage caused by the chemotherapy agent paclitaxel.[492] *Precautions: May lower blood sugar. Certain components in maitake enhance immune function while other components suppress immune function. Be sure to speak with your oncologist before using, and use only under the guidance of a trained practitioner.*

MYCOPHYTO COMPLEX

This commercial dietary supplement is a blend of several medicinal mushrooms: Agaricus blazei, Cordyceps, Turkey tail, Reishi, Maitake, Polyporus umbellatus, and a few other ingredients. Although this supplement is not manufactured specifically for cancer, in vitro studies have shown MycoPhyto Complex to suppress triple negative breast cancer metastasis.[493] *Precautions: View the precautionary statements under each individual type of mushroom listed on the product's label.*

OYSTER MUSHROOM
Pleurotus ostreatus

Oyster mushrooms are another popular culinary ingredient which can be found in some supermarkets and are commonly seen in Asian cuisine. Oyster mushrooms have been shown to induce tumor cell death. Some studies have shown that these mushrooms are especially effective for inhibiting the growth of colon cancer and ER+/PR+ breast cancer cells.[494] Simply add the mushrooms to your favorite cuisine. *Precautions: Some individuals may experience increased sensitivity to mold when eating oyster mushrooms on a regular basis. Ingesting large amounts of whole oyster mushroom may cause abdominal pain. If you choose to grow your own oyster mushrooms be sure to wear a face mask as some individuals may develop sensitivity to the mushroom's spores.*

PROSTACAID

ProstaCaid is a commercial dietary supplement made by the same company as the MycoPhyto Complex mentioned above. ProstaCaid's ingredients include medical mushrooms such as Reishi, Turkey Tail, and Song Gen, as well as a special blend of other herbs, vitamins, and minerals. In vitro studies have shown ProstaCaid to suppress the growth of hormone refractory prostate cancer cells.[495] *Precautions: Be sure to read the ingredients listing carefully to ensure you are not allergic to any of*

---

491 *Maitake Beta-glucan Enhances Therapeutic Effect and Reduces Myelosuppression and Nephrotoxicity of Cisplatin in Mice* (Masuda, 2009)

492 *Maitake Beta-glucan Promotes Recovery of Leukocytes and Myeloid Cell Function in Peripheral Blood from Paclitaxel Hematotoxicity* (Lin, 2010)

493 *Novel Medicinal Mushroom Blend Suppresses Growth and Invasiveness of Human Breast Cancer Cells,* (Jiang, 2010)

494 *Pleurotus ostreatus Inhibits Proliferation of Human Breast and Colon Cancer Cells Through p53-dependent as Well as p53-independent Pathway.* (Jedinak, 2008)

495 *ProstaCaid Inhibits Tumor Growth in a Xenograft Model of Human Prostate Cancer.* (Jiang,, 2012)

them. Because this blend contains so many ingredients I strongly recommend that you review the ingredients with your oncologist to be sure none of them will work against your prescribed treatments.

REISHI
Ganoderma lucidum/ G. sinensis

Also known as Ling Zhi. Reishi is known for reducing tumor blood vessel formation by inhibiting the production of VEGF and it also contains triterpene compounds which inhibit metastasis. Reishi tea is rather bitter, so many patients opt for injections or commercial supplements instead. In vitro studies have shown reishi to decrease the development of pre-cancerous lesions in the colon,[496] as well as inhibit ovarian cancer while enhancing the efficacy of cisplatin.[497] Terpenes isolated from this mushroom have been shown to reduce kidney damage caused by the chemotherapy agent cisplatin.[498] Reishi also has significant action against cancer-related fatigue in breast cancer patients who are undergoing endocrine therapy.[499] *Precautions: Only use under competent professional supervision as too much of this agent can cause major harm to your liver. May cause diarrhea. Is a blood thinner. Reishi mushroom spores may increase levels of glycoprotein CA72-4, a protein seen in cancers such as gastrointestinal, ovarian, uterine, and lung, therefore I do not recommend growing these at home.*

SCALY WOOD MUSHROOM
Agaricus sylvaticus /Agaricus blazei

This mushroom is typically found in Brazil and Japan and may go by other names such as sun mushroom, kawarihiratake, and himematsutake. In various medical studies this mushroom has shown potential for inhibiting blood vessel formation within tumors as well as inducing cancer cell death. A Brazilian study gave patients scaly wood mushrooms as part of their diet after bowel cancer surgery, finding that patients who received the mushrooms had a better quality of life compared to patients who did not receive the mushrooms. The benefits included: improved mood, reduced pain, reduced insomnia, increased appetite, reduced bowel problems, and reduced nausea.[500] One study involving breast cancer patients who were supplemented with this mushroom during chemotherapy experienced decreased nausea (80%) and improved appetite (20%).[501] *Precautions: Use of this mushroom*

---

496 *A Water-soluble Extract from Culture Medium of Ganoderma lucidum Mycelia Suppresses the Development of Colorectal Adenomas.* (Oka, 2010)

497 *Ganoderma lucidum Exerts Anti-tumor Effects on Ovarian Cancer Cells and Enhances Their Sensitivity to Cisplatin.* (Zhao, 2011)

498 *Prevention of Cisplatin Induced Nephrotoxicity by Terpenes Isolated from Ganoderma lucidum Occurring in Southern Parts of India.* (Pillai, 2011)

499 *Spore Powder of Ganoderma Lucidum Improves Cancer-Related Fatigue in Breast Cancer Patients Undergoing Endocrine Therapy: A Pilot Clinical Trial* (Hong Zhao, et al 2012)

500 *Life quality of post surgical patients with colorectal cancer after supplemented diet with agaricus sylvaticus fungus.*(Costa Fortes, 2010)

501 *Effect of Agaricus sylvaticus supplementation on nutritional status and adverse events of chemotherapy of breast cancer: A randomized, placebo-controlled, double-blind clinical trial*

may cause liver problems in some patients therefore you should use only with your physician's supervision. This mushroom may lower blood sugar levels. Has strong estrogenic properties; check with your oncologist before consuming if you are undergoing any kind of hormonal treatments or have an estrogen-fueled cancer.

SHIITAKE
Lentinula edodes

Shiitake mushrooms, another popular culinary ingredient, contains a water soluble substance called lentinan which is known to have strong medicinal qualities. Due to its water solubility be sure to consume the broth/water that is released during the cooking process. If instead you take commercial lentinan supplements be sure to drink a full glass of water with your supplement to encourage the absorption of the lentinan into your system. In the medical field lentinan is used as an intravenous anti-cancer drug with anti-tumor properties. Clinical studies have associated lentinan with a higher survival rate, higher quality of life and lower recurrence of cancer. According to the Memorial Sloan Kettering Cancer Center, lentinan has been shown to increase the repair of DNA damage in bone marrow caused by paclitaxel treatments, induces cell death in stomach cancers (especially when used in tandem with the chemotherapy agents docetaxel and cisplatin), and increases cancer cell death in bladder cancers (especially when combined with the chemotherapy agent gemcitabine). It has also been shown to enhance the effects of paclitaxel against lung cancer. Simply cook the mushrooms in with your favorite cuisine. *Precautions: May cause bloating, diarrhea or other digestive disturbances. May cause eosinophilia – an increase in certain types of white blood cells – therefore consult with your oncologist first if you are being treated for leukemia. Lentinan may enhance the effects of AZT. Some individuals may be sensitive to the lentinans.*

SONG GEN
Phellinus linteus

This mushroom, also known as black hoof mushroom, is usually found growing on elm, willow and mulberry trees. Studies have shown that using song gen with doxorubicin treatments increased the number of prostate cancer cells killed,[502] enhances the effects of doxorubicin induction of cell death in lung cancer,[503] inhibits the metastasis of melanoma cancers, [504] and halts an enzyme used by breast cancer cells to create new blood vessels in the tumors.[505] Two case studies report patients with liver cancer experiencing shrinkage of tumors after treatment with song gen: (1) A man with liver metastasis to his skull and other bones refused standard treatment (except for radiation) and used the mushroom with significantly positive results.[506] (2)

(Valadares, 2013)

502 *Phellinus linteus Sensitizes Apoptosis Induced by Doxorubicin in Prostate Cancer* (Collins, 2006)

503 *Modulation of Lung Cancer Growth Arrest and Apoptosis by Phellinus linteus.* ((Guo, 2007)

504 *Acidic Polysaccharide from Phellinus linteus Inhibits Melanoma Cell Metastasis by Blocking Cell Adhesion and Invasion* (Han, 2006).

505 **British Journal of Cancer**, *Press Release, April 15, 2008*

506*Spontaneous Regression of a Large Hepatocellular Carcinoma with Skull Metastasis* (Nam, 2005)

A man with liver cancer metastasized to the lung was reported to experience tumor regression after using *P. linteus* extracts for one month even though he did not receive conventional treatments.[507] Another case study reports a patient with metastasized hormone refractory prostate cancer (for which there is no distinctive treatment) who experienced a dramatic regression in the disease after using song gen extracts.[508] *Precautions: May worsen certain autoimmune disorders, causing blisters and itching. Do not use without competent professional oversight.*

TURKEY TAIL
Coriolus versicolor/ Tramates v. / Polyporus v. / Polystictus v.

Turkey Tail mushrooms are the source of Polysaccharide-K, (a.k.a. PSK, a.k.a. Krestin) and Polysaccharide Peptide (PSP) – substances known to be strong anti-cancer agents. Clinical studies have shown PSK is effective against acute nonlymphocytic leukemia when used as maintenance therapy.[509] PSK has also been shown to enhance the action of monoclonal antibodies against colon cancer,[510] slow the deterioration of patients with non-small cell lung cancer,[511] and reduce recurrence/increase survival rates of colorectal cancer patients taking oral Tegafur and Uracil.[512] One Japanese study saw that patients who underwent surgery for gastric cancers who were followed with treatment using Mitomycin-C, Futraful, and PSK enjoyed a significantly longer survival rate.[513] PSP has also been shown to induce cell death in promyelocytic leukemia cells.[514] In vitro studies have observed that extracts of Turkey Tail mushroom reduces the growth of B-cell lymphoma and promyelocytic leukemia cells.[515] It has also been shown that Turkey Tail enhances the effects of camptothecin against promyeolocytic leukemia cells.[516]

---

507 *A Case of Spontaneous Regression of Hepatocellular Carcinoma with Multiple Lung Metastases.* (Kojima, 2006)

508 *Dramatic Remission of Hormone Refractory Prostate Cancer Achieved with Extract of the Mushroom Phellinus linteus.* (Shibata, 2004)

509 *A Randomized Trial of Chemoimmunotherapy of Acute Nonlymphocytic Leukemia in Adults Using a Protein-bound Polysaccharide Preparation.* (Ohno, 1984)

510 *Activation of Peritoneal Macrophages by Polysaccharopeptide from the Mushroom Coriolus versicolor.* (Liu, 1993)

511 *Coriolus versicolor Polysaccharide Peptide Slows Progression of Advanced Non-small Cell Lung Cancer* (Tsang, 2003)

512 *Adjuvant Immunochemotherapy with Oral Tegafur/Uracil Plus PSK in Patients with Stage II or III Colorectal Cancer: A Randomized Controlled Study.* (Ohwada, 2004)

513 *Postoperative Adjuvant Immunochemotherapy with Mitomycin-C, Futraful, and PSK for Gastric Cancer. An Analysis of Data on 579 Patients Followed for Five Years.* (Niimoto, 1988)

514 *The Cell Death Process of the Anticancer Agent Polysaccharide-peptide (PSP) in Human Promyelocytic Leukemic HL-60 Cells.* (Yang, 2005)

515 *Cytotoxic Activities of Coriolus versicolor (Yunzhi) Extract on Human Leukemia and Lymphoma Cells by Induction of Apoptosis.* (Lau, 2004)

516 *Polysaccharopeptides Derived from Coriolus versicolor Potentiate the S-phase Specific Cytoxicity of camptothecin (CPT) on Human Leukemia HL-60 Cells,* (Wan, 2010)

Chapter 13
SPIRITUAL GUIDANCE

The idea of using spirituality, religion, and prayer for healing is often met with skepticism and suspicion, however research has shown that using spirituality, religion, and prayer as complementary treatment is significantly effective for patient health. The evidence is plentiful and I cannot list all of it in this book, however I will cite a few examples:

- A review of ninety studies investigating both hands-on prayer and distance prayer revealed that 70% of the clinical studies and 62% of the laboratory studies reported positive results when using prayer for healing.[517]
- One study observed that patients who used meditation prayer had greater reduction in anxiety, greater increase in mood, and experienced nearly twice the pain tolerance than those who used regular meditation.[518]
- One randomized, double-blind study involved a total of 393 hospitalized heart patients who were given standard treatment. Roughly one half were given intercessory prayer performed off the hospital campus while the remainder had no prayer performed for them. After treatment was finished it was noted that the group who were prayed for experienced less need for for ventilators, antibiotics, and diuretics compared to the non-prayer group.[519]
- One double blind study tested the effects of distance healing through prayer on forty patients suffering from advanced AIDS. Patients and distance healers never met. After six months it was found that the patients who were given distance healing experienced reduced severity of illness, reduced need for doctor appointments, reduced need for hospitalization, and increased improvement in mood.[520]
- Dartmouth Medical Center found that in a pool of 232 patients undergoing open heart surgery the six month post-surgical survival rate was fourteen times *higher* in religious/social patients in comparison to the patients who were non-religious/social.[521]
- A study involving North Carolina residents followed a group of 4,000 elderly people for six years, observing that study subjects who attended religious services on a regular basis had a significantly lower rate of death compared to those who attended infrequently.[522]

---

517 *A Systematic Review of the Quality of Research on Hands-on and Distance Healing; Clinical and Laboratory Results.* (Crawford, 2003)

518 *Is spirituality a critical ingredient of meditation? Comparing the effects of spiritual meditation, secular meditation, and relaxation on spiritual, psychological, cardiac, and pain outcomes.* (Wachholtz, 2005)

519 *Positive therapeutic effects of intercessory prayer in a coronary care unit population.* (Byrd, 1988)

520 *A Randomized Double-blind Study of the Effect of Distant Healing in a Population with Advanced AIDS. Report of a Small Scale Study.* (Sicher, 1998)

521 *Lack of Social Participation or Religious Strength and Comfort as Risk Factors for Death After Cardiac Surgery in the Elderly.* (Oxman, 1995)

522 *Does religious attendance prolong survival? A six-year follow-up study of 3,968 older adults.*

- One study examined the results of more than 5,000 patients over a twenty-eight year period and found that those who attended religious services on a frequent basis experienced lower mortality rates than those who attended religious services infrequently or not at all.[523]

- A Harvard study[524] analyzed the religious service attendance habits of 75,000 women within a sixteen year period and found the following observations: **(1)** Those who attended religious services more than once per week experienced a 33% lower mortality rate, those attending once per week had a 26% lower mortality rate, and those attending less than weekly had a 13% lower mortality rate. **(2)** Women who attended services regularly were less likely to be tobacco users, experienced lower rates of depression, and were more likely to have a strong social network – all factors which are known to promote better health.

- An Israeli study published in 1993 followed more than 10,000 Israeli men over a twenty-three years to monitor for heart disease and observed that those who were the most religious were 20% less likely to die from coronary disease compared to the less religious men.[525]

- One study showed that when a group of cancer patients were divided in half based on their levels of pain and fatigue the patients who were more spiritually inclined tended to experience a high quality of life in comparison to the patients who were less spiritual.[526]

Clearly, spirituality, religion, and prayer are directly linked with one's response during illness and therefore these are essential pieces in holistic therapy. Do not feel foolish about feeding this need when you are battling cancer; it is more foolish to ignore it.

When you are looking for something to address your spiritual needs keep in mind that there is no single way to go about it; each individual has his or her own specific needs which vary, and that is okay. Because there is such variety among individuals this chapter will cover an assortment of spiritually-centered methods that may be useful to you. I strongly encourage you to explore the following options:

Guided Imagery: Guided imagery comes in eight different forms – one of which is guided spiritual imagery. This form of imagery uses pre-recorded scripts which are intended to guide you into focusing on sensing the presence of God, Jesus, and the angels, and your spiritual connections with them. Although you can have a professional guided imagery therapist create a recording for you, you may also ask your pastor or other church member to help you create one. Alternatively, you can search for faith-based guided spiritual imagery scripts online and self-record those which resonate with you. When choosing guided imagery keep in mind that it is meant to soothe and create peace within you, therefore this should never be a rushed

(Koenig, 1999)

523 *Frequent Attendance at Religious Services and Mortality Over 28 Years.* (Strawbridge, 1997).

524 **Harvard Health Publications**, Harvard Medical School, *Attending Religious Services Linked to Longer Lives, Study Shows*, published July 2016

525 *Factors Predictive of Long-term Coronary Heart Disease Mortality Among 10,059 Male Israeli Civil Servants and Municipal Employees.* (Goldbourt, 1993)

526 *The Role of Religion/Spirituality for Cancer Patients and Caregivers* (Weaver, 2004)

session. Plan to spend at least half an hour or more in a quiet location free from distractions.

Communing With God: This is very similar to guided imagery except you are not being guided by a script; instead you are letting your mind and emotions freely commune with God without any particular focal point. Choose a quiet location free from distractions such as a grassy field, a calm body of water, a secluded wooded area, a candle lit room, a church prayer room, etc. wherever you feel safe and relaxed. Like guided imagery this should not be a rushed session; give yourself at least half an hour or more for this spiritual communion.

Scriptural Meditation: This is a session in which you focus on a single Scriptural passage that strengthens you mentally, emotionally, and spiritually. Set aside a specific time to meditate on your chosen passage several times per week. Alternatively you may choose a few passages and rotate them throughout the week. If you are unsure which passages you want to use do not hesitate to ask your congregational leader or believing friends for suggestions; alternatively you may wish to perform an internet search for Scriptures to meditate on. Some Scriptural passages that are popular include Psalm 19, Psalm 23, Psalm 25, Psalm 46, Matthew 5 3-10, and Revelation 21:1-7.

Affirmation Prayers: These are short, personal prayers you repeat to yourself during times of trouble, pain, depression, etc. These are usually about one sentence in length and are designed to help you keep your spiritual focus during tough times. Repeat your chosen affirmation prayer as often as you need. Some examples of affirmation prayers are (references taken from the CSB):[527]

- Psalm 23:4 "Even when I go through the darkest valley, I fear no danger, for you are with me; your rod and Your staff – they comfort me."
- 2 Corinthians 4:17 "For our momentary light affliction is producing for us an absolutely incomparable eternal weight of glory."
- Matthew 11:28 "Come to me, all of you who are weary and burdened, and I will give you rest."
- Romans 8:16 "The Spirit himself testifies together with our spirit that we are God's children."
- Nahum 1:7 "The LORD is good, a stronghold in a day of distress; he cares for those who take refuge in him."
- Philippians 4:13 "I am able to do all things through him who strengthens me."
- Psalm 56:3 "When I am afraid, I will trust in You."

Prayer Circles: This is when you schedule a get-together with other people for the purpose of praying for each other as a means to strengthen one another spiritually. You can arrange prayer circles with your friends, neighbors, family members, or with other people in your church congregation or cancer support group. Whenever possible try to schedule your prayer circles at regular intervals (weekly, monthly, daily, whatever works for you and your circle). Prayer circles are usually done in person,

---

527 Scripture quotations marked CSB have been taken from the Christian Standard Bible®, Copyright © 2017 by Holman Bible Publishers. Used by permission. Christian Standard Bible® and CSB® are federally registered trademarks of Holman Bible Publishers.

but if distance or illness is in the way you can also have your prayer groups meet over a conference call, video chat, or group chat. God is not limited by location.

Anointing With Oil: The practice of anointing the sick with oil, sometimes known as "Unction of the Sick," is based on the Scripture at James 5:14. which says (CSB) "Is anyone among you sick? He should call for the elders of the church, and they are to pray over him, anointing him with oil in the name of the Lord." Many congregations perform this service so do not hesitate to ask.

Prayer Partner: This is a small version of the prayer circle – choose a singular person who is willing to make time for the two of you to pray together. Again try to schedule this on a regular basis, depending upon what works for you and your prayer partner. And again, if distance or illness is a problem you can perform your prayer sessions over the phone, video chat, or text; God is not limited by location.

Hospital Chaplains: If you find yourself hospitalized for any reason, whether or not it is related to your cancer, it is worth your while to schedule time for the hospital chaplain to come visit you in your room. If you are dependent upon a health care proxy to make your decisions for you be sure your proxy knows ahead of time that you will want chaplain visits scheduled during hospital stays. Chaplains can lend a listening ear, pray with you, and read Scripture to you as you wish.

Individual Prayer: Never neglect your own personal one-on-one time with God. Schedule a time each day in which you can quietly pray in the privacy of your home and mind. Speak to your Heavenly Father, open up all your thoughts, feelings and fears. He is your Heavenly Father and He cares about what you have to say.

Hands-on Prayer: This is when a group of fellow believers lay their hands gently on you as they pray for you and your situation. This can be done in the context of a prayer circle, with a prayer partner, during a church service, or with a hospital chaplain.

Pastoral Counseling: Many congregations have health ministries and/or visitation ministers who go out visiting congregation members who are unable to get out due to illness. Sign up to be on the visitation list and be sure any health ministers know that you have a situation and that you need your spiritual concerns met. Even in smaller congregations where there are no such ministries you may still schedule time to speak with your pastor in order to obtain such healing.

Weekly Worship Services: Attending your local weekly worship services is another good way to feed your spirituality. If you are unable to attend the weekly service in person ask if the congregation streams their services online or via telephone so you can still "attend." If not, ask if they post pre-recorded sermons and services on their website so that you can still view and hear them on a regular basis. It is also worth noting that many churches have a bus ministry in which they will come and take you to the services and back if you are otherwise unable to get out.

Shawl and Blanket Ministries: Many churches offer ministries in which members make hand-made items to give to those who are ill, injured, or in recovery. One such ministry is known as the Prayer Shawl Ministry, in which the members knit or crochet shawls while praying over the person who the shawl is being made for. Other similar ministries may make lap quilts, fleece blankets, or other items for the same purpose. Contact your local church to sign up to receive one of these heart warming gifts.

Christian Media: Another way to feed your spirituality during your battle with cancer is to listen to Christian-based media. Whether it is your local Christian radio station, a television pastor, a roster of Christian-based YouTube videos, or listening to sermons online through Christian websites, make a list of the programs and media that speak to your heart and schedule regular time to listen or view.

Daily Devotional Reading: These are short, one-page Bible themed collections of writing usually in book or magazine form. You can either buy daily devotional books at local bookstores (or online), subscribe to online daily devotionals which can be emailed or sent to your phone, or subscribe to monthly daily devotional magazines through the mail.[528]

Christian Music: Sometimes music is the perfect thing to feed one's spirit. This can run the gamut of listening to Gregorian chants, traditional church hymns, contemporary Christian music, traditional gospel, southern gospel, choir music, and more. If your energy allows, you may even choose to join and actively participate in a church singing choir or bell choir in order to get closer to the music. If you play a musical instrument, and if your energy allows, offer to play music at your church services, congregation picnics, and other ministries.

What if you are someone who has no connection to a local congregation, thus limiting your access to some of the above-mentioned methods? It is never too late to get involved with a local congregation of your choice. The Internet has simplified the "church search" process so that you can check out your local congregations to determine which of them can meet your needs. Browse the listings, check their websites, and do not hesitate to make phone calls or send out an email if you have questions about their ministries and services. Let them know what you need, whether it is transportation to the services, attendance via telephone or live-stream, anointing with oil, etc. Even if a certain congregation may not have what you need they may be able to direct you to a congregation who can. If you happen to live in an area without sufficient church options (such as rural areas) you may also choose to search for online faith-based chat groups or message forums to seek the spiritual healing you need.

Do not fear, for I am with you; do not be afraid, for I am your God. I will strengthen you; I will help you; I will hold on to you with my righteous right hand.
– Isaiah 41:10 (CSB)

---

528 Popular devotionals received by mail include (but are not limited to): Our Daily Bread, The Upper Room, Today, etc.

APPENDIXES

APPENDIX 1
CYP3A4 Inducers

Some of these drugs may be known by other names. Speak with your prescribing physicians if you have any questions or if you do not see your medication on this list.

Alfentanil	Alprazolam	Amlodipine
Amprenavir	Aprepitant	Armodafinil
Aripiprazole	Astemizole	Atorvastatin
Avasimibe	Boceprevir	Bosentan
Buspirone	Carbamazepine	Chlorpheniramine
Cilostazol	Cocaine	Codeine-N-demethylation
Cyclosporine	Dapsone	Dexamethasone
Dextromethorphan	Diazepam	Diltiazem
Docetaxel	Efavirenz	Eplerenone
Ergotamine	Erythromycin	Estradiol
Etravirine	Ethosuximide	Fentanyl
Finasteride	Glucocorticoids	Griseofulvin
Haloperidol	Hydrocortisone	Imatinib
Indinavir	Irinotecan	Lercanidipine
Levomethadyl acetate	Lidocaine	Lovastatin
Methadone	Midazolam	Modafinil
Nafcillin	Nateglinide	Nelfinavir
Nevirapine	Nifedipine	Nisoldipine
Nitrendipine	Omeprazole	Ondansetron
Oxcarbazepine	Paclitaxel	Phenobarbital
Phenylbutazone	Phenytoin	Pioglitzaone
Pimozide	Prednisone	Primidone
Progesterone	Propanolol	Quetiapine
Quinidine	Quinine	Rifabutin
Rifampin	Rufinamide	Risperidone
Ritonavir	Rofecoxib	Romidepsin

Saquinavir	Salmeterol	Sildenafil
Simvastatin	Sirolimus	Sorafinib
Sulfadimidine	Sulfinpyrazone	Sunitinib
Tacrolimus	Telaprevir	Telithromycin
Temsirolimus	Testosterone	Trazodone
Triazolam	Troglitazone	Vemurafenib
Verapamil	Vincrcristine	Zaleplon
Ziprasidone		

Take note that sometimes a single medication may contain some ingredients which are inducers and some which are inhibitors. Because the above table is not a comprehensive list I advise you to speak with your prescribing physicians.

APPENDIX 2
CYP3A4 Inhibitors

Some of these drugs may be known by other names. Speak with your prescribing physicians if you have any questions if you do not see your medication on this list.

Amiodarone	Amprenavir	Atazanavir
Boceprevir	Cimetidine	Ciprofloxacin
Clarithromycin	Cyclosporine	Danazol
Delavirdine	Diltiazem	Efavirenz
Ethinyl	Ezetimibe	Fluconazole
Fluoxetine	Fluvoxamine	Gestodene
Imatinib	Indinavir	Isoniazid
Itraconazole	Ketoconazole	Methylprednisolone
Mibefradil	Miconazole	Mifepristone
Nefazodone	Nelfinavir	Nicardipine
Nifedipine	Norethindrone	Norfloxacin
Norfluoxetine	Oxiconazole	Posaconazole
Prednisone	Quinine	Ranolazine
Ritonavir	Roxithromycin	Saquinavir
Sertraline	Telaprevir	Telithromycin
Troleandomycin	Verapamil	Voriconazole
Zafirlukast	Zileutin	

Take note that sometimes a single medication may contain some ingredients which are inducers and some which are inhibitors. Because the above table is not a comprehensive list I advise you to speak with your prescribing physicians.

APPENDIX 3
Timing of Chemotherapy Agents

In the past decade researchers have discovered that, due to the body's circadian rhythm, the efficacy of chemotherapy treatments can be increased simply by adjusting the time of day in which they are given. The circadian rhythm is your body's 24 hour cycle based on stimulation from the daylight/nighttime cycle. This rhythm dictates your natural wake/sleep cycle, timing of hormones released throughout the day, brain wave activity, and cell regeneration.

Just like normal body cells, cancer cells also need to regenerate themselves, especially when enduring the severe damage caused by radiation and chemotherapy agents being used to destroy them. Researchers have found that if chemotherapy is given during the time of the circadian rhythm when these cancer cells are *least* able to repair themselves they are more easily destroyed.

Dr. Yosef Yarden and his team of researchers at the Weizmann Institute of Science in Israel found that the body's normal day-time release of certain steroids would bind to the EGF[529] receptors on cancer cells effectively blocking chemotherapy agents from attaching instead. Using mice they discovered that administering chemotherapy agents during the sleep phase resulted in significantly smaller tumors after only one week, in comparison to the mice that were given the agent during the awake time. And, not only were the night-administered tumors smaller, but they also showed less infiltration of blood vessels in the tumors, indicating the tumors were much weaker than the day-treated tumors.

Other studies have shown that another factor in timing is due to the ebb and flow of certain enzymes throughout the 24 hour cycle which tend to hinder the efficacy of some chemotherapy agents. This enzyme system is known as nucleotide excision repair – its job is to repair particular kinds of DNA damage in body cells. Dr. Aziz Sancar and his research team at the North Carolina School of Medicine studied this problem and found the following: Using mouse models the team discovered that DNA repair occurred six times faster in the morning hours than in the evening hours. Dr. Sancar stated *"By hitting cancer cells with chemotherapy at a time when their ability to repair themselves is minimal, you should be able to maximize the effectiveness and minimize the side effects of treatment."* Since many chemotherapy agents work by causing DNA damage to the cancer cells, timing one's treatments to work when this enzyme is less active is a crucial element in beating the disease.[530]

There have been many studies performed regarding the timing of chemotherapy agents and these have yielded important information. For example:

- ***Ovarian cancer:*** Giving doxorubicin early in the morning is less toxic and allows white blood cell counts to recover a week sooner than when it is given

---

529 EGF = **E**pidermal **G**rowth **F**actor, a protein which stimulates cell production.

530 In many cases slow growing tumors tend to be more synchronized with the normal circadian rhythm and fast growing tumors tend to deviate from the normal rhythm.

in the evening. Patients who are given a tandem treatment of doxorubicin in the morning and cisplatin twelve hours later, in the evening, experience a 44% five-year survival rate, whereas patients given the reverse treatment (cisplatin in the morning and doxorubicin in the evening) experience a mere 11% five-year survival rate.

- *Bladder cancer*: Patients with metastatic bladder cancer who were given doxorubicin in the morning and cisplatin in the evening experienced a significant shrinkage of their tumors with some tumors disappearing altogether. Patients with localized bladder cancer undergoing this same regimen experienced a significant decrease in metastasis.

- *Renal cell cancer*: The majority of patients with advanced disease given a continuous infusion of fluorodeoxyuridine (a.k.a. FUDR) from 3pm-9pm experienced a significant shrinkage in tumors and more than one year of stability.[531] Patients also experienced less severe side effects.

Chemotherapy agents in certain classes are associated with optimal times to be given; this is why it is important to know which classes your chemotherapy agents are listed under. If you do not know this information do not hesitate to ask your oncologist. The general rule of thumb for some of the different classes is as follows:

- *Alkylating agents*, which break DNA strands, should be taken in the evening hours.
- *Anti-metabolite agents*, which break DNA, tend to do best when taken during the late evening or just before going to bed for the night.
- *Corticosteroids* and *interferons* tend to do best when given either just at the time of awakening or just before sleeping.
- *Platinum-based agents* tend to do best when taken between 4pm -6pm

By following a schedule which works with your circadian rhythm your chemotherapy agents can work harder and better for you; in some cases this may mean decreasing your chemotherapy dosages which translates into a decrease in side effects.

If you are a night-shift worker then this timing will be completely different for you, since are living and working against your body's natural rhythm. This means that if you cannot get your work schedule changed to day shift then you need to create an artificial day/night cycle to stabilize your circadian rhythm. Here are some ways to accomplish this:

- During your overnight waking hours stay in brightly lit areas; do not dim the lights in your work space if at all possible. Keep yourself in at least 10-12 hours of bright light during your overnight hours whenever possible.

---

531 "Stability" denotes that, although some cancer is still detected, it does not increase or spread.

- Do not consume energy drinks or caffeinated products for six hours before sleep time. If you go to sleep at 8a.m. Then discontinue the beverages at 2a.m.
- Do not eat anything for at least three hours before sleep; the increased energy your body needs for digestion may prevent the "slow down" you need for sleep. Therefore, an 8a.m. sleep time requires that you do not eat after 5a.m.
- If you must commute home in the bright light of morning try wearing dark sunglasses on your way home to prevent the daylight from overstimulating your brain.
- Do not drink any fluids for at least one hour before sleep so that you will not be disrupted with the urge to urinate during your sleep time.
- Darken your bedroom with black shades and dark, heavy curtains. If you must, tape the sides of the shades to the window frame to prevent daylight from "leaking" in.
- Turn off your phone so that it does not disturb your sleep.
- Try to schedule any daytime appointments during the very early morning hours or in the late afternoon whenever possible to reduce interruption of sleep.
- Keep your light/dark schedule, even on your days off, as much as possible. The less you deviate from this schedule the more stable your circadian rhythm will remain.

APPENDIX 4
Acupuncture

The origin of acupuncture is based on the principles of energy medicine taught in the philosophical ideas of Chinese Taoism. It began with ancient Chinese physicians who believed that good health is dependent upon a balanced flow of vital energy known as qi or chi (both pronounced as "*chee*"). It has been taught that qi energy flows through the body along linear pathways called meridians, and each meridian is associated with a particular organ or organ system. The idea is that, if something blocks or hinders the flow of qi then illness results; this flow must be restored in order to restore one's health. In order to restore this flow the ancient physicians developed a method of skin stimulation using sharpened stone and carved bone tools. Over time these tools were modified into the hair-thin needles that are used in modern acupuncture today. Today, most practitioners of Traditional Chinese Medicine in the United States also perform acupuncture treatments.

Many Christians may find themselves uncomfortable with the relationship of acupuncture to Taoism and thus avoid it completely as a therapy. The problem is that this is "throwing the baby out with the bath water" so to speak. Although medical science does not prove the existence of qi it has actually proven the existence, structure, and activity of the *meridians*. For example:

In the 1960's a team of North Korean researchers discovered the primo vascular system[532] – a system of ducts in the body running along meridian lines. The fluid in these channels were not associated with either blood or lymph. Later, in the 1970's Dr. Liu, a licensed acupuncturist at the University of North Carolina, discovered that certain points along the meridian lines were associated with areas of dense nerve bundles, suggesting a mechanism of response.[533]

In 1992 French researchers performed tests to visualize the meridians by injecting radioactive isotopes along the meridian lines in volunteers. When following the isotopes for several centimeters it was observed that the isotopes within the acupoints actually followed the meridian pathways, whereas the non-acupoint isotopes simple diffused from the injection site in a circular formation. It was also observed that insertion of an acupuncture needle in a distant point on a marked meridian they were following would result in an increased flow rate of the isotope.[534]

During another study at the University of York, using MRI imaging, it was found that acupuncture elicits a unique response in the brain that is different from responses associated with pain.[535] In a similar study, researchers at the Hull York Medical School investigated the relationship between the brain's neural responses

---

532 *Evidence-Based Complimentary and Alternative Medicine,* "*50 Years of Bong-Han Theory and 10 Years of Primo Vascular System,*" Volume 2013

533 *The American Journal of Chinese Medicine*, "*The Correspondence Between Some Motor Points and Acupuncture Loci*", Volume 3, Issue 4, 1975

534 *Nuclear Medicine and Acupuncture Massage Transmission*, Pierre de Vernejoul, Pierre Albarede, Jean-Claude Darras (1992)

535 *Brain Imaging of Acupuncture: Comparing Superficial With Deep Needling* (MacPherson, 2008)

with the sensation of deqi[536] during acupuncture. Like the University of York study, this study also used MRI scans to document brain response and found that pain response and deqi response were significantly different in the brain, according to the MRI records.[537]

Like all other sensory information, stimulation signals from acupuncture needles sprint to the brain directly through the spinal cord.[538] When the input from the spinal cord reaches the brain it immediately activates areas of the brain devoted to the reception of, and response to, sensory stimulation.[539] Oftentimes the brain's response is to release various amounts of neurotransmitters such as endorphins (which reduce pain), neuropeptides (which can reduce nausea and vomiting) and serotonin (which can reduce fatigue) depending upon the stimulation it receives. Although there is still much to learn about the relationship between acupuncture and the brain it is known that this basic process is what makes acupuncture work. Clearly, a patient does not need to subscribe to the philosophies of Taoism in order to derive therapeutic benefit as science shows there is a real, physical mechanism that makes acupuncture therapy work.

When seeking an acupuncturist, be sure he or she is a board certified licensed professional. Also make sure your practitioner is aware of any health issues that may need special care including locations of solid tumors, recent surgeries, radiation treatments, and lymphedema.

536"Deqi" (pronounced *deh-kee'*) is described in different ways among patients. Descriptions include: Heaviness, numbness, dull pain, soreness, achiness, warmth, tingling, fullness, coolness, electric, etc. Some describe deqi as non-painful sensations traveling among acupoints. Although this happens with a vast majority of acupuncture patients (up to 85%), it does not happen with all patients.

537 *Acupuncture Needling Sensation: The Neural Correlates of Deqi Using fMRI* (Ashgar, 2010)

538 The spinal cord attaches directly into your brain and is the main conduit for delivering sensory information to your brain. This is why the spinal cord branches out into so many nerve pathways throughout your body.

539 *Neural mechanism underlying acupuncture analgesia* (Zhi-Qi Zhao, 2008)

APPENDIX 5
Aromatherapy

In its most basic definition aromatherapy is the use of aromatic essential oils for inhalation-based therapy. Essential oils are highly concentrated substances derived from the fruits, flowers, seeds, leaves, roots, and bark of various plants. Because these substances are so highly concentrated they are too strong for internal use; this means you should never introduce them into your eyes, ears, nose, mouth, rectum, vagina or penis, even in a diluted form.

During inhalation with aromatherapy the microscopic molecules of the agent are small enough to pass through your nasal membranes directly into your circulatory system. From there the molecules are carried to your brain which houses your limbic system; a network of nerves and neural tissues which control emotions, drive, motivation, long-term memory, adrenaline response, and your sense of smell. Different aromatherapy agents stimulate different areas of the limbic system. When deciding to use aromatherapy agents check with your physician first before using this method if you have asthma, COPD, emphysema, pulmonary sclerosis, or any other lung problems.

An alternative way to use an aromatherapy agent as a direct inhalant is to mix it with a carrier oil and use it topically as an aromatic massage oil. Because the oils are so strong you must dilute them in a carrier oil (mineral oil or vegetable oil) in order to reduce the risk of skin irritations. A typical dilution is 12 drops of essential oil to 2 tablespoons (30 ml) of carrier oil. Topical applications can be in the form of a massage oil, a cold compress, lotion, or salve. Do not use on open or broken skin, fresh surgical sites, areas on or around solid tumors, areas being treated with topical chemotherapy, radiation, light, or heat therapy without consulting with your physician first.

Take note that some people may tell you that that certain oils such as tea tree oil or lavender oil are gentle enough to use without dilution (known as "neat"). I disagree: There have been cases in which users have applied them undiluted and then some time later developed a rapid sensitization to the substance, causing severe skin issues. Once you've become sensitized you are sensitized for life, whether you use it full strength or with a carrier oil. Since no one can know if or when she will become sensitized the best way to avoid this mistake is to play it safe by always using a carrier oil.

At this point I should bring up a topic that will invariably be mentioned to you if you have an estrogen-fueled cancer: There is this idea that tea tree oil and lavender oil have estrogenic properties and therefore ER+ cancer patients should steer clear of them. This idea originated from a study led by Dr. Derek Henley, Ph. D. which was published in 2007. This study suspected that lavender oil and tea tree oil, which were found to have weak estrogenic effect *in vitro*,[540] had caused three young boys exposed

---

[540]"*In vitro*" means in a test tube or other container outside the human body. In vitro tests do not involve living beings such as laboratory animals (*in vivo* studies) or human studies (clinical trials).

to these oils to experience breast growth even though their exposure was limited to normal use of commercial products.[541] The study stated *"On the basis of the three case reports and the in vitro studies, we suspect that repeated topical application of over-the-counter products containing lavender oil or tea tree oil was the cause of [breast growth] in the three patients."* and then went on to recommend *"Until epidemiologic studies are performed to determine the prevalence of gynecomastia associated with exposure to lavender oil and tea tree oil, we suggest that the medical community should be aware of the possibility of endocrine disruption and should caution patients about repeated exposure to any products containing these oils."*

Henley's study was criticized due to its assumptions, erroneous information and lack of scientific data: The study claimed tea tree oil is *"chemically similar"* to lavender oil, which it is not. The study gave no details regarding the other ingredients in the commercial products used by the boys, no details about the composition of the oils tested in vitro, and no attempts were made to evaluate the levels of oils in the commercial products in question. It was also found that none of the constituents in tea tree oil that penetrate human skin are estrogenic and that the oil actually inhibits the ability of other substances to penetrate the skin. Although lavender oil is shown to be weakly estrogenic *in vitro*, there is no scientific evidence showing that the oil reacts the same when metabolized and processed in a living person. Also, the report does not mention whether the boys were exposed to any pesticides, (some of which have estrogenic effects) or whether they were exposed to other estrogenic substances such as phthalates or parabens that are common in many cosmetic products. In short, the study contained only superficial information and virtually none of the ideas or suppositions contained within were substantiated.[542] In spite of Henley's study being so heavily flawed and incomplete, the idea that these oils are estrogenic continue to circulate.

Since a living being metabolizes and processes substances in ways that *in vitro* tests do not, an *in vitro* result cannot be translated as having the same exact results in a living being without being tested first.

541 *The New England Journal of Medicine*, Feb.1, 2007, 356, pp.479-485 *"Prepubertal Gynecomastia Linked to Lavender and Tea Tree Oils"*, Derek. V. Henley, Ph. D

542 *"Neither Lavender Oil Nor Tea Tree Oil Can Be Linked to Breast Growth In Young Boys"*, Robert Tisserand., world renowned aromatherapist and massage therapist. This article gives valid scientific sources and reference information too numerous to include in this chapter.

APPENDIX 6
Guided Imagery [543]

Also known as "visualization" and "mental imagery," guided imagery is known for helping reduce anxiety and depression and at times may also help increase a patient's immune function.

Although guided imagery can be a very useful tool, what can it do for patients undergoing chemotherapy? In one review of several studies it was observed that the use of guided imagery with cancer patients increased patients' sense of well-being and comfort.[544] Another study involving a mixed group of breast and prostate cancer patients (492 patients total) found a significant reduction in the levels of stress hormones and anxiety in those who underwent guided imagery therapy.[545] In two different studies it was observed that guided imagery increases the immune function in some cancer patients.[546] [547] There have also been studies to investigate the use of guided imagery to cope with cancer-related pain and treatment-related nausea, but results among the studies are currently inconsistent.

There are various methods of guided imagery/visualization, and everyone responds differently to each one. Methods may include sessions which focus on visualizing healthy interactions in your body cells, the flow of natural energy in your body, imagery that evokes pleasant mood or thoughts, and meditation on one's connection with God, among other methods.

Guided imagery is more than simple imagination or pleasant thoughts. Oftentimes it can include your other senses such as hearing, smell, and touch. For example, during a session you may listen to a recording of twittering birds or gentle music. You can burn incense, use aromatherapy, or lie out in a field to stimulate your sense of smell. For your sense of touch you can pet your purring cat, wear something soft and comforting, or have a second person massage you during your session.

Of course, you may not need to use *all* of your senses in a session; in fact that may be too overwhelming. Do only what feels right and comfortable for *you*. What works for one person may not necessarily work for another. You may choose to focus on one sense, or combine a few senses together; there is no wrong answer, it is whatever works best for you.

---

543 Take note: Anyone can label him or herself as a guided imagery therapist without special licensing. Therefore, look for a therapist who has had formal training by a reputable practitioner or educational program.

544 *A systematic review of guided imagery as an adjuvant cancer therapy.* (Roffe, 20050

545 *A Randomized Controlled Trial for the Effectiveness of Progressive Muscle Relaxation and Guided Imagery as Anxiety Reducing Interventions in Breast and Prostate Cancer Patients Undergoing Chemotherapy.* (Charalambous, 2015)

546 **Journal of Psychosomatic Research,** Dec. 2002, Vol.53, No.6, pp.1131-1137, "*The effect of hypnotic-guided imagery on psychological well-being and immune function in patients with prior breast cancer*", Anthony C. Bakke

547 **The Breast**, Feb. 2009, Vol.18, Issue 1, pp.17-25, "*Immuno-modulatory effects of relaxation training and guided imagery in women with locally advanced breast cancer undergoing multimodality therapy*" Oleg Eremin

The following are the eight primary methods of guided imagery with a very brief description of each:

Method	Description
Feeling State	Visualizes happy, peaceful, positive thoughts and emotions.
End State	Visualizes the realization of a goal: Winning a race, hitting a perfect singing note, finishing a project, etc.
Energetic imagery	Visualizes the inner energy in your body flowing unblocked and unhindered.
Cellular imagery	Visualizes the healthy interaction of body cells such as the uptake of oxygen into blood cells, intake of nutrients, etc.
Physiological imagery	Visualizes the healing processes in the body, such as the shrinkage of tumors or the action of immune cells taking charge.
Metaphoric imagery	Visualization in symbols instead of reality, such as imagining the tumor as an enemy army being destroyed by soldiers with weapons.
Psychological imagery	Visualizes psychologically soothing situations such as being surrounded by friends and loved ones.
Spiritual imagery	Visualizes your connection with God, Jesus, and the angels.

APPENDIX 7
Music Therapy

Music therapy is more than just a simple session of listening to your favorite tunes. Depending upon the circumstances a music therapy program may include any combination of musical instruments, tones, vocal exercises, and physical movement. This can include (but is not limited to) exercises in song writing, creating musical notes with instruments, moving rhythmically to instrumental compositions, writing sheet music, relaxing to a specific combination of tones, singing, and more. Some music therapy programs may be created for singular patients and other programs may be more socialized, such as a drum circle or a choir. Because each patient's needs are unique there is no "one-size-fits-all" therapy. A patient is not required to have musical ability in order to participate in music therapy.

Numerous studies have shown that listening to music causes your brain to release special neurotransmitters known to improve mood, sleep, and pain response. Some of the neurotransmitters released in response to music include *dopamine*,[548] a chemical associated with feelings of reward and pleasure, *serotonin*,[549] known for reducing depression and regulating sleep, *endorphins*,[550] known for improving mood and reducing pain signals, and *melatonin*,[551] which is known to regulate sleep and mood.

Another positive effect of music is its ability to help reduce the levels of the stress hormone, cortisol, in the patient's system.[552] Cortisol is produced as a response to stress in order to help the body cope with the stress. When a patient is under a prolonged period of stress (such as with major illnesses like cancer) the continual production of cortisol can cause prolonged healing times, cause digestive issues, increase blood pressure, and cause insomnia and depression. By reducing cortisol levels music therapy can help restore a patient's stamina, sleep, and well-being. One particular pilot study headed by Sarah J. I. Burns, RMT (registered music therapist) showed strong evidence of increased immune function in cancer patients who received music therapy.[553] Another study which followed 111 healthy volunteers participating in group drumming sessions showed an increase in the activity of

---

548 *Anatomically distinct dopamine release during anticipation and experience of peak emotion to music* (Salimpoor, 2011)

549 *Changes of the neurotransmitter serotonin but not of hormones during short time music perception* (Evers, 2000)

550 *Performance of music elevates pain threshold and positive affect: implications for the evolutionary function of music.* (Dunbar, 2012)

551 *Music therapy increases serum melatonin levels in patients with Alzheimer's disease.* (Kumar, 1999)

552 **EXCLI Journal**, 2012, Vol. 11, pp.556-565, "*The Effect of Music on the Level of Cortisol, Blood Glucose, and Physiological Variables in Patients Undergoing Spinal Anesthesia*" Elaheh Mottahedian Tabrizi, et al

553 **Alternative Therapies**, Jan. 2001, Vol. 7, No.1, "*A Pilot Study Into the Therapeutic Effects of Music Therapy at a Cancer Help Center*" Sarah J. I. Burns, RMT

Natural Killer cells and other immune cells in their systems.[554] Since immune function can be compromised during cancer therapy, this is a very important finding in medicine. One particularly comprehensive study showed that the benefits of music therapy include reduction in the use of painkilling medications, sedation medications, cancer pain, and anxiety along with significant improvements in blood pressure and heart rate.[555] A Cochrane review of 30 cancer studies involving nearly 1,800 participants found that music therapy helps to improve mood and quality of life in cancer patients while also reducing anxiety and pain.[556]

Music therapy is a recognized health service much like physical therapy or occupational therapy, with the main difference being that this type of therapy uses music as the therapeutic medium. Music therapists are board-certified professionals who have successfully completed a music therapy program through an accredited school. Their educational curriculum includes classes in psychology, behavioral sciences, disabilities, and general studies as well as music. They are also trained in evaluating patients' needs as well as how to develop individualized treatment plans.

554 *Alternative Therapies*, Jan. 2001, Vol. 7, No.1, "*Composite Effects of Group Drumming Music Therapy on Modulation of Neuroendocrine-Immune Parameters in Normal Subjects*" Barry B. Bittman, et al

555 *Music therapy as an adjuvant therapeutic tool in medical practice: an evidence-based summary* (Mattei, 2013)

556 *Cochrane Library*, Aug. 2011, "*Music interventions for improving psychological and physical outcomes in cancer patients*" J. Bradt, et al

www.ingramcontent.com/pod-product-compliance
Lightning Source LLC
Chambersburg PA
CBHW081124170526
45165CB00008B/2538